GINGER AND MAGNESIUM BOOK

"The Supreme Guide to Restoring Balance, Relieving Pain, and Boosting Energy for Dynamic Living, including Delicious Recipes and Meal Plans to Intensify Your Well-being"

Dr. Lukas Loewe

Copyright © 2024

Dr. Lukas Loewe

TABLE OF CONTENTS

Dr. Lukas Loewe

CHAPTER 1:
INTRODUCTION TO GINGER AND MAGNESIUM

1.1 Understanding the Health Benefits of Ginger

Ginger, a fragrant and flavorful root, is not only a staple in cuisines worldwide but also holds a long-standing reputation for its medicinal properties. Its health benefits range from soothing digestive issues to reducing inflammation and even combating nausea. Let's delve into the intricate ways ginger influences human health and psychology.

- *Digestive Health:*

One of the most well-known benefits of ginger lies in its ability to support digestive health. It aids in digestion by stimulating the production of enzymes that break down food and promote smooth movement through the digestive tract. This can be particularly beneficial for individuals experiencing indigestion, bloating, or discomfort after meals.

Research suggests that ginger can help alleviate symptoms of gastrointestinal distress, such as nausea and vomiting, which can have a significant impact on psychological well-being. For example, individuals undergoing chemotherapy or experiencing morning sickness during pregnancy often find relief from these symptoms by consuming ginger. By reducing physical discomfort, ginger may also alleviate associated feelings of anxiety or distress, contributing to an overall sense of well-being.

- *Anti-inflammatory Properties:*

Inflammation is a natural response of the immune system to injury or infection, but chronic inflammation can contribute to various health issues, including arthritis, heart disease, and certain mental health conditions. Ginger contains potent anti-inflammatory compounds, such as gingerol, which have been shown to reduce inflammation in the body.

By alleviating inflammation, ginger may indirectly benefit psychological health. Studies have suggested a link between inflammation and mental health disorders such as depression and anxiety. By reducing systemic inflammation, ginger may

help mitigate symptoms of these conditions, promoting a more balanced mood and improved psychological resilience.
Pain Relief:

Beyond its anti-inflammatory properties, ginger also possesses analgesic effects, meaning it can help reduce pain. This makes it a valuable natural remedy for individuals dealing with conditions such as osteoarthritis, menstrual cramps, or migraines. By modulating pain perception, ginger may not only alleviate physical discomfort but also positively influence psychological well-being.

The connection between pain and psychological health is well-established. Chronic pain conditions can significantly impact mood, sleep quality, and overall quality of life, leading to feelings of frustration, irritability, or even depression. By providing relief from pain, ginger may help alleviate these negative psychological effects, promoting a greater sense of comfort and emotional balance.

1.2 The Importance of Magnesium in Human Physiology

Magnesium is an essential mineral that plays a crucial role in numerous physiological processes throughout the body. From supporting muscle function to regulating blood pressure and maintaining bone health, magnesium is involved in a wide array of functions that directly impact physical and psychological well-being.

- Muscle Function and Relaxation:

One of the primary roles of magnesium is its involvement in muscle function and relaxation. Magnesium works in concert with calcium to regulate muscle contractions and nerve impulses. Adequate magnesium levels help muscles relax after contraction, preventing cramps, spasms, and tension.

The relationship between muscle relaxation and psychological state is profound. Muscle tension is a common physical manifestation of stress and anxiety. Individuals experiencing chronic stress may develop tightness or stiffness in their muscles, contributing to feelings of discomfort and agitation. By

Dr. Lukas Loewe

promoting muscle relaxation, magnesium may help alleviate these physical symptoms and induce a sense of calmness and relaxation, which can positively impact psychological well-being.

- *Regulation of Stress Response:*
Magnesium plays a vital role in the body's stress response system, influencing the activity of the hypothalamic-pituitary-adrenal (HPA) axis and the release of stress hormones such as cortisol. Chronic stress can deplete magnesium levels in the body, creating a cycle where stress further exacerbates magnesium deficiency, leading to potential negative consequences for both physical and psychological health.

Studies have shown that magnesium supplementation may help modulate the body's stress response, reducing the release of cortisol and promoting a more balanced physiological reaction to stressors. By supporting healthy stress adaptation, magnesium may mitigate the negative psychological effects of chronic stress, such as anxiety, depression, or burnout.

- *Neurotransmitter Regulation:*
Magnesium is involved in the regulation of neurotransmitters, the chemical messengers that facilitate communication between neurons in the brain. Magnesium ions are necessary for the proper function of receptors involved in neurotransmitter release and signal transduction.

Optimal neurotransmitter function is essential for maintaining mood stability, cognitive function, and overall psychological well-being. Imbalances in neurotransmitter levels or function have been implicated in various mental health disorders, including depression, anxiety, and bipolar disorder. By supporting neurotransmitter regulation, magnesium may help promote mental clarity, emotional stability, and resilience to stressors.

1.3 Synergistic Effects of Ginger and Magnesium on Health
While ginger and magnesium each offer unique health benefits on their own, their combined effects can be even more potent when used together. The synergy between these two natural

Dr. Lukas Loewe

remedies can enhance their individual properties and provide comprehensive support for overall health and well-being.

- *Digestive Health and Nutrient Absorption:*

Both ginger and magnesium play crucial roles in supporting digestive health and nutrient absorption. Ginger stimulates digestion by promoting the production of digestive enzymes and enhancing gastric motility, while magnesium helps regulate muscle function in the digestive tract and supports the absorption of nutrients.

By combining ginger and magnesium, individuals may experience improved digestion and nutrient assimilation, which can have far-reaching effects on physical and psychological health. Proper digestion ensures that essential nutrients are absorbed efficiently, providing the body and brain with the fuel needed for optimal function. Additionally, a healthy digestive system has been linked to improved mood and cognitive function, as gut health influences the production of neurotransmitters and inflammatory markers.

- *Stress Reduction and Relaxation:*

Both ginger and magnesium possess properties that promote relaxation and stress reduction, albeit through different mechanisms. Ginger contains compounds with anti-inflammatory and analgesic effects that can help alleviate physical tension and discomfort, while magnesium supports muscle relaxation and regulates the body's stress response system.

By combining ginger's calming effects with magnesium's ability to promote muscle relaxation and regulate stress hormones, individuals may experience enhanced relaxation and stress resilience. This synergistic approach to stress management can have profound effects on psychological well-being, helping individuals cope more effectively with daily stressors and maintain a greater sense of balance and equanimity.

Dr. Lukas Loewe

- Inflammation Modulation and Mood Regulation:

Inflammation and mood are intricately linked, with chronic inflammation contributing to the development and exacerbation of mood disorders such as depression and anxiety. Both ginger and magnesium possess anti-inflammatory properties that can help modulate inflammatory processes in the body.

By combining ginger's anti-inflammatory compounds with magnesium's regulatory effects on neurotransmitters and stress hormones, individuals may experience comprehensive support for mood regulation and emotional well-being. This synergistic approach targets multiple pathways implicated in mood disorders, offering a holistic strategy for promoting mental health and resilience.

In conclusion, the combination of ginger and magnesium offers a powerful synergy that can support overall health and well-being from both physical and psychological perspectives. By understanding the individual benefits of these natural remedies and their complementary effects, individuals can harness their synergistic potential to optimize health outcomes and enhance quality of life.

Dr. Lukas Loewe

CHAPTER 2:
GINGER: NATURE'S HEALING ROOT

2.1 History and Cultural Significance of Ginger

Ginger, known scientifically as Zingiber officinale, is a flowering plant native to Southeast Asia that has been cultivated for thousands of years for its culinary and medicinal properties. Its history and cultural significance span diverse civilizations and continents, reflecting its widespread popularity and esteemed reputation.

Historical Roots: The use of ginger dates back to ancient times, with evidence of its cultivation and consumption found in ancient Chinese, Indian, and Middle Eastern civilizations. In China, ginger has been documented in writings dating back to the 4th century BCE, where it was prized for its medicinal properties and included in traditional herbal remedies.

Similarly, in ancient India, ginger was revered as a sacred plant and was considered a valuable trade commodity along the Spice Route. It was used not only in cooking but also in Ayurvedic medicine for its digestive and anti-inflammatory properties. In the Middle East, ginger was highly regarded for its aromatic and medicinal qualities, with historical texts referencing its use in culinary dishes and therapeutic preparations.

Cultural Significance: Throughout history, ginger has held symbolic and cultural significance in various societies. In ancient Rome, ginger was associated with wealth and luxury, often used in elaborate feasts and banquets hosted by the elite. It was also used as a symbol of hospitality, with hosts offering gingerbread or ginger-infused treats to guests as a gesture of welcome and goodwill.

In many Asian cultures, ginger is deeply ingrained in culinary traditions and is considered a staple ingredient in dishes ranging from savory stir-fries to sweet desserts. Its pungent flavor and warming properties are believed to stimulate the appetite and aid digestion, making it an indispensable component of traditional cuisine.

Dr. Lukas Loewe

In addition to its culinary uses, ginger has played a role in various cultural practices and rituals. In some cultures, ginger is believed to possess protective qualities and is used in rituals to ward off evil spirits or bring good luck. In others, it is used ceremonially in religious rites or as a symbol of purity and healing.

2.2 Nutritional Composition and Active Compounds in Ginger

Ginger is packed with nutrients and bioactive compounds that contribute to its therapeutic properties and health benefits. From vitamins and minerals to potent phytochemicals, the nutritional composition of ginger makes it a valuable addition to a balanced diet and a potent remedy in traditional and modern medicine.

Vitamins and Minerals: Despite its small size, ginger is rich in essential vitamins and minerals that play vital roles in maintaining overall health. It contains significant amounts of vitamin C, an antioxidant that supports immune function and helps protect cells from damage caused by free radicals. Additionally, ginger provides small amounts of vitamins B3 (niacin) and B6 (pyridoxine), which are involved in energy metabolism and nervous system function.

In terms of minerals, ginger is particularly notable for its manganese content, with just one teaspoon of ground ginger providing approximately 5% of the recommended daily intake. Manganese is essential for bone health, wound healing, and the metabolism of carbohydrates, proteins, and fats. Ginger also contains small amounts of potassium, magnesium, and phosphorus, which contribute to various physiological processes in the body.

Active Compounds: The therapeutic properties of ginger can be attributed to its rich array of bioactive compounds, including gingerol, shogaol, and paradol. These compounds possess antioxidant, anti-inflammatory, and antimicrobial properties, making ginger an effective natural remedy for a wide range of health conditions.

Gingerol is perhaps the most well-studied compound in ginger and is responsible for its characteristic pungent flavor and spicy aroma. It exhibits potent antioxidant activity, helping to neutralize free radicals and protect cells from oxidative damage. Additionally, gingerol has been shown to have anti-inflammatory effects, which may help alleviate pain and reduce the risk of chronic diseases such as heart disease and cancer.

Shogaol is another bioactive compound found in ginger, formed when gingerol is dehydrated during the drying or cooking process. Like gingerol, shogaol possesses antioxidant and anti-inflammatory properties and has been studied for its potential therapeutic effects on conditions such as nausea, vomiting, and inflammatory bowel disease.

Paradol, a lesser-known compound in ginger, has recently gained attention for its pharmacological properties, including its potential anti-cancer effects. Studies have shown that paradol may inhibit the growth and proliferation of cancer cells by inducing apoptosis (cell death) and suppressing tumor formation. While more research is needed to fully understand its mechanisms of action, paradol holds promise as a novel therapeutic agent in cancer treatment.

2.3 Therapeutic Uses of Ginger in Traditional and Modern Medicine

Ginger has been used medicinally for centuries in various cultures around the world, prized for its diverse therapeutic properties and wide-ranging health benefits. From alleviating nausea to reducing inflammation and improving digestive health, ginger continues to be a popular natural remedy in both traditional and modern medicine.

Digestive Health: One of the most well-known uses of ginger is its ability to alleviate digestive discomfort and promote gastrointestinal health. Ginger stimulates the production of digestive enzymes and enhances gastric motility, helping to alleviate symptoms such as indigestion, bloating, and flatulence. It is particularly effective in easing nausea and vomiting associated with motion sickness, pregnancy, or chemotherapy.

Research suggests that ginger may also help alleviate symptoms of gastrointestinal disorders such as irritable bowel syndrome (IBS) and inflammatory bowel disease (IBD). Its anti-inflammatory and anti-spasmodic effects may help reduce intestinal inflammation and alleviate abdominal pain and discomfort, improving overall quality of life for individuals with these conditions.

Anti-inflammatory and Pain Relief: Ginger's potent anti-inflammatory properties make it a valuable remedy for reducing pain and inflammation throughout the body. It has been studied for its effectiveness in relieving pain associated with conditions such as osteoarthritis, rheumatoid arthritis, and muscle soreness.

Studies have shown that ginger extract can significantly reduce pain and improve joint function in individuals with osteoarthritis, making it a promising natural alternative to conventional pain medications. Its analgesic effects are thought to be mediated by its ability to inhibit the production of inflammatory cytokines and prostaglandins, which contribute to pain and inflammation.

In addition to its anti-inflammatory effects, ginger has been shown to enhance the efficacy of nonsteroidal anti-inflammatory drugs (NSAIDs) when used in combination, allowing for lower doses and reduced risk of side effects. This synergistic effect may make ginger a valuable adjunct therapy for individuals seeking natural pain relief with fewer adverse effects.

Immune Support and Respiratory Health: Ginger contains compounds with immune-boosting properties that can help support the body's natural defense mechanisms and protect against infections. Its antimicrobial and antiviral effects make it particularly effective in combating respiratory infections such as the common cold and flu.

Research has shown that ginger extract can inhibit the growth of respiratory pathogens such as influenza virus and respiratory syncytial virus (RSV), reducing the severity and duration of respiratory symptoms. Its warming properties may also help soothe sore throats and relieve congestion, making ginger a popular remedy for respiratory ailments.

Furthermore, ginger's anti-inflammatory effects may help alleviate symptoms of allergic rhinitis (hay fever) by reducing inflammation in the nasal passages and airways. By modulating immune responses and reducing inflammatory markers, ginger may help alleviate symptoms such as nasal congestion, sneezing, and itching associated with allergic reactions.

In summary, ginger is a versatile and potent natural remedy with a rich history of use in traditional medicine and a growing body of scientific evidence supporting its therapeutic benefits. From alleviating digestive discomfort to reducing inflammation and supporting immune function, ginger offers a holistic approach to health and wellness that aligns with human psychology's innate desire for natural solutions and holistic approaches to healing.

CHAPTER 3:
MAGNESIUM: THE MIGHTY MINERAL

3.1 Sources and Bioavailability of Magnesium

Magnesium is a vital mineral that the human body requires for various physiological functions, yet many people do not consume enough of it through their diet. Understanding the sources and bioavailability of magnesium is essential for ensuring adequate intake and promoting optimal health.

- *Sources of Magnesium*

Magnesium is naturally present in many foods, with some sources being more abundant than others. Here are some common dietary sources of magnesium:

1. **Leafy green vegetables:** Spinach, kale, Swiss chard, and other leafy greens are excellent sources of magnesium. These vegetables contain high levels of magnesium due to their chlorophyll content, which is rich in magnesium ions.
2. **Nuts and seeds:** Almonds, cashews, peanuts, pumpkin seeds, and sunflower seeds are all good sources of magnesium. These foods provide not only magnesium but also healthy fats, protein, and fiber, making them nutritious snacks or additions to meals.
3. **Whole grains:** Whole grains such as brown rice, quinoa, oats, and whole wheat are rich in magnesium. Consuming whole grains instead of refined grains ensures a higher intake of magnesium and other essential nutrients.
4. **Legumes:** Beans, lentils, chickpeas, and other legumes are rich sources of magnesium and provide additional benefits such as protein, fiber, and vitamins.
5. **Seafood:** Certain types of seafood, such as salmon, mackerel, halibut, and tuna, contain significant amounts of magnesium. Incorporating seafood into your diet can help boost your magnesium intake while providing essential omega-3 fatty acids.
6. **Dairy products:** Dairy products like milk, yogurt, and cheese contain magnesium, although the amounts may vary depending on processing and fortification.

Dr. Lukas Loewe

7. **Dark chocolate:** Dark chocolate with a high cocoa content is a surprisingly rich source of magnesium. Enjoying a square or two of dark chocolate as a treat can contribute to your daily magnesium intake.

- *Bioavailability of Magnesium*

Bioavailability refers to the extent to which a nutrient is absorbed and utilized by the body after consumption. Several factors influence the bioavailability of magnesium from dietary sources:

1. **Nutrient interactions:** Certain nutrients and dietary components can enhance or inhibit magnesium absorption. For example, vitamin D facilitates magnesium absorption, while phytic acid and dietary fiber can impair absorption.
2. **Food processing:** Processing methods such as cooking, soaking, and fermentation can affect the bioavailability of magnesium in foods. For instance, boiling vegetables may leach magnesium into the cooking water, reducing its availability in the final dish.
3. **Individual factors:** Factors such as age, gender, genetics, and overall health can influence how efficiently the body absorbs and utilizes magnesium. Individuals with certain medical conditions or taking certain medications may have altered magnesium absorption rates.
4. **Magnesium salts:** Magnesium is commonly available in various supplemental forms, including magnesium oxide, magnesium citrate, magnesium glycinate, and magnesium chloride. These different forms have varying levels of bioavailability, with magnesium citrate and glycinate generally being more readily absorbed than magnesium oxide.

To enhance magnesium absorption from dietary sources, it's essential to consume diverse and balanced diet rich in magnesium-rich foods while paying attention to factors that may affect bioavailability.

3.2 Functions of Magnesium in the Body

Magnesium plays a crucial role in numerous physiological processes throughout the body, contributing to overall health and well-being. From supporting muscle function to regulating blood pressure and maintaining bone density, magnesium is involved in a wide array of functions that are essential for human health.

Muscle Function: Magnesium is necessary for proper muscle function, including muscle contraction and relaxation. It works in conjunction with calcium to regulate muscle contractions by activating and deactivating muscle fibers. Adequate magnesium levels help muscles relax after contraction, preventing cramps, spasms, and stiffness.

The importance of magnesium in muscle function extends beyond skeletal muscles to include smooth muscles found in organs such as the heart, blood vessels, and gastrointestinal tract. Proper magnesium levels are essential for maintaining cardiovascular health, regulating blood pressure, and supporting digestive function.

Energy Metabolism: Magnesium plays a crucial role in energy metabolism, serving as a cofactor for over 300 enzymatic reactions involved in the synthesis and breakdown of ATP (adenosine triphosphate), the body's primary energy currency. Magnesium is required for the activation of enzymes involved in glycolysis, the citric acid cycle, and oxidative phosphorylation, processes that generate ATP from carbohydrates, fats, and proteins.

By facilitating energy production at the cellular level, magnesium ensures that cells have the energy needed to perform essential functions, maintain homeostasis, and support overall metabolic health. Inadequate magnesium levels can impair energy metabolism, leading to fatigue, weakness, and decreased physical performance.

Bone Health: Magnesium is essential for maintaining bone health and density, working in concert with calcium, vitamin D, and other minerals to support bone formation and remodeling. Approximately 60% of the body's magnesium is stored in the bones, where it helps regulate calcium and phosphate levels and promotes the formation of hydroxyapatite, the mineral matrix of bone tissue.

Studies have shown that low magnesium intake is associated with decreased bone mineral density and an increased risk of osteoporosis and fractures. Adequate magnesium levels are essential for optimizing bone health throughout life, from childhood and adolescence, when bone formation is at its peak, to older adulthood, when bone density begins to decline.

Nervous System Function: Magnesium plays a crucial role in nervous system function, influencing neurotransmitter release, neuronal signaling, and neuromuscular transmission. It acts as a modulator of calcium channels and NMDA receptors, which are involved in synaptic transmission and synaptic plasticity.

Magnesium deficiency has been implicated in various neurological and neuropsychiatric disorders, including migraine headaches, anxiety, depression, and epilepsy. Studies have shown that magnesium supplementation can help alleviate symptoms of migraine headaches and improve mood and cognitive function in individuals with depression and anxiety disorders.

Cardiovascular Health: Magnesium is essential for maintaining cardiovascular health, regulating cardiac rhythm, and supporting vascular function. It helps maintain the electrical stability of cardiac cells and modulates the activity of ion channels involved in cardiac conduction and contraction.

Low magnesium levels have been associated with an increased risk of cardiovascular diseases such as hypertension, arrhythmias, and coronary artery disease. Magnesium supplementation has been shown to lower blood pressure, improve endothelial function, and reduce the risk of cardiovascular events in individuals with hypertension and other risk factors.

Immune Function: Magnesium plays a vital role in immune function, influencing the activity of immune cells and the production of cytokines and antibodies. It helps regulate inflammatory responses and oxidative stress, contributing to the body's defense against infections and diseases.

Studies have shown that magnesium deficiency can impair immune function and increase susceptibility to infections. Conversely, adequate magnesium levels support immune function and enhance the body's ability to mount an effective immune response.

In summary, magnesium is a mighty mineral with diverse functions that are essential for human health and well-being. From supporting muscle function and energy metabolism to maintaining bone health and cardiovascular function, magnesium plays a vital role in numerous physiological processes throughout the body. Ensuring an adequate intake of magnesium through diet and supplementation is crucial for promoting optimal health and reducing the risk of deficiency-related health problems.

3.3 Common Deficiency Symptoms and Health Implications

Magnesium deficiency, also known as hypomagnesemia, is a common yet often overlooked nutritional deficiency that can have significant health implications. Understanding the symptoms and consequences of magnesium deficiency is essential for identifying and addressing potential deficiencies to promote optimal health and well-being.

Symptoms of Magnesium Deficiency

Magnesium deficiency can manifest with a wide range of symptoms affecting various systems in the body. Common signs and symptoms of magnesium deficiency include:

1. **Muscle cramps and spasms:** Magnesium plays a crucial role in muscle function and relaxation. Deficiency can lead to muscle cramps, spasms, and stiffness, particularly in the legs and feet.
2. **Fatigue and weakness:** Magnesium is involved in energy metabolism and ATP production. Deficiency can result in fatigue, weakness, and reduced physical performance.

3. **Nausea and vomiting:** Magnesium deficiency can affect gastrointestinal function, leading to symptoms such as nausea, vomiting, and loss of appetite.
4. **Irregular heartbeat:** Magnesium is essential for maintaining normal cardiac rhythm and conduction. Deficiency can result in palpitations, arrhythmias, and other cardiovascular problems.
5. **Mood changes:** Magnesium plays a role in neurotransmitter regulation and mood stabilization. Deficiency may contribute to symptoms such as irritability, anxiety, and depression.
6. **Headaches and migraines:** Magnesium deficiency has been implicated in the pathogenesis of headaches and migraines. Supplementing with magnesium may help alleviate symptoms and reduce the frequency and severity of migraines.
7. **Insomnia and sleep disturbances:** Magnesium plays a role in regulating neurotransmitters and promoting relaxation. Deficiency may interfere with sleep quality and contribute to insomnia and sleep disturbances.

- *Health Implications of Magnesium Deficiency*

Magnesium deficiency can have significant health implications and may increase the risk of various acute and chronic health problems. Some of the health implications of magnesium deficiency include:

1. **Cardiovascular disease:** Low magnesium levels have been associated with an increased risk of hypertension, coronary artery disease, and arrhythmias. Magnesium deficiency may contribute to endothelial dysfunction, vascular inflammation, and oxidative stress, promoting the development of cardiovascular disease.
2. **Osteoporosis and bone health:** Magnesium is essential for maintaining bone density and bone mineralization. Deficiency can impair bone formation and increase the risk of osteoporosis and fractures, particularly in older adults.
3. **Metabolic syndrome and diabetes:** Magnesium plays a role in glucose metabolism and insulin sensitivity. Deficiency may contribute to insulin resistance, impaired glucose

tolerance, and the development of metabolic syndrome and type 2 diabetes.

4. **Neurological disorders:** Magnesium deficiency has been implicated in various neurological and neuropsychiatric disorders, including migraine headaches, anxiety, depression, and epilepsy. Supplementing with magnesium may help alleviate symptoms and improve neurological function.

5. **Muscle and joint problems:** Magnesium deficiency can lead to muscle cramps, spasms, and weakness, as well as joint pain and stiffness. Adequate magnesium levels are essential for maintaining muscle and joint health and preventing musculoskeletal problems.

6. **Immune dysfunction:** Magnesium plays a role in immune function and inflammation regulation. Deficiency may impair immune responses and increase susceptibility to infections and inflammatory diseases.

7. **Hormonal imbalances:** Magnesium is involved in the synthesis and metabolism of hormones such as insulin, cortisol, and thyroid hormones. Deficiency may disrupt hormonal balance and contribute to various hormonal imbalances and related health problems.

In summary, magnesium deficiency is a common nutritional problem with significant health implications. Recognizing the signs and symptoms of magnesium deficiency and addressing potential deficiencies through dietary changes, supplementation, and lifestyle modifications is essential for promoting optimal health and reducing the risk of deficiency-related health problems.

CHAPTER 4:
INCORPORATING GINGER AND MAGNESIUM INTO DAILY LIFE

4.1 Practical Tips for Adding Ginger to Your Diet

Ginger is a versatile and flavorful ingredient that can be easily incorporated into various dishes and beverages to reap its numerous health benefits. Whether fresh, dried, or in powdered form, ginger adds a delightful zing to both sweet and savory recipes.

Here are some practical tips for adding ginger to your diet:

1. **Ginger Tea:** One of the simplest ways to enjoy the benefits of ginger is by making ginger tea. To prepare ginger tea, thinly slice fresh ginger root and steep it in hot water for 5-10 minutes. You can enhance the flavor by adding a squeeze of lemon juice or a drizzle of honey. Enjoy ginger tea as a soothing beverage any time of day, especially during cold weather or when feeling under the weather.

2. **Smoothies and Juices:** Adding fresh or powdered ginger to smoothies and juices is an excellent way to incorporate this potent ingredient into your diet. Simply toss a few slices of fresh ginger or a teaspoon of powdered ginger into your blender along with your favorite fruits and vegetables. Ginger pairs well with citrus fruits like oranges and lemons, as well as tropical fruits like pineapple and mango.

3. **Stir-fries and Curries:** Ginger adds depth and complexity to stir-fries and curries, enhancing their flavor and aroma. Finely mince or grate fresh ginger and sauté it with garlic, onions, and other aromatics before adding vegetables, protein, and sauces. Ginger pairs particularly well with ingredients like garlic, soy sauce, coconut milk, and chili peppers, creating delicious Asian-inspired dishes.

4. Baked Goods: Ginger adds warmth and spice to baked goods such as cookies, cakes, and muffins. Ground ginger, ginger powder, or crystallized ginger can be incorporated into recipes to impart a subtle gingery flavor. Try adding ground ginger to oatmeal cookies, gingerbread cake, or pumpkin muffins for a festive and flavorful twist.

5. **Salad Dressings and Marinades:** Ginger can also be used to make flavorful salad dressings and marinades. Combine fresh ginger, garlic, soy sauce, rice vinegar, sesame oil, and honey to create a tangy and aromatic dressing for salads or grilled vegetables. You can also use ginger in marinades for meats, tofu, or seafood to infuse them with flavor before cooking.

6. **Pickled Ginger:** Pickled ginger, also known as sushi ginger or gari, is a popular condiment in Japanese cuisine. It is made from thinly sliced young ginger that has been pickled in a mixture of vinegar, sugar, and salt. Pickled ginger is often served alongside sushi or sashimi to cleanse the palate between bites and aid digestion. You can also use pickled ginger as a garnish for salads, rice bowls, or noodle dishes.

Incorporating ginger into your diet is easy and delicious, allowing you to enjoy its numerous health benefits while adding flavor and excitement to your meals and beverages. Whether you prefer it fresh, dried, or pickled, ginger is a versatile ingredient that can elevate any dish or drink with its unique and invigorating taste.

4.2 Strategies for Increasing Magnesium Intake Naturally

Magnesium is an essential mineral that plays a crucial role in numerous physiological processes in the body, yet many people do not consume enough magnesium through their diet alone. Fortunately, there are several strategies you can employ to increase your magnesium intake naturally:

1. **Eat Magnesium-Rich Foods:** One of the most effective ways to boost your magnesium intake is by incorporating more magnesium-rich foods into your diet. Some excellent dietary sources of magnesium include leafy green vegetables (such as spinach, kale, and Swiss chard), nuts and seeds (such as almonds, cashews, and pumpkin seeds), whole grains (such as brown rice, quinoa, and oats), legumes (such as beans, lentils, and chickpeas), and seafood (such as salmon, mackerel, and halibut). By prioritizing these foods in your meals and snacks, you can increase your magnesium intake naturally.

2. **Choose Whole Foods:** Whole foods tend to be richer in magnesium compared to processed and refined foods. Therefore, choosing whole, minimally processed foods over highly processed options can help boost your magnesium intake. Opt for whole grains instead of refined grains, whole fruits and vegetables instead of fruit juices and canned fruits, and whole nuts and seeds instead of nut butters and roasted snacks. By focusing on whole foods, you can ensure that you're getting a more nutrient-dense diet that includes plenty of magnesium-rich options.

3. **Cook with Herbs and Spices:** Certain herbs and spices are surprisingly good sources of magnesium and can be used to add flavor to your meals while increasing your magnesium intake. For example, dried herbs like basil, coriander, and dill, as well as spices like cumin, mustard seeds, and black pepper, contain notable amounts of magnesium. Incorporating these herbs and spices into your cooking can not only enhance the taste of your dishes but also contribute to your overall magnesium intake.

4. **Soak and Sprout Grains, Nuts, and Seeds:** Soaking and sprouting grains, nuts, and seeds can enhance their magnesium bioavailability by reducing the presence of phytic acid, an antinutrient that can inhibit mineral absorption. Phytic acid is found in the outer layers of grains, nuts, and seeds and can bind to minerals like magnesium, preventing them from being absorbed by the body. By soaking and sprouting these foods before consumption, you can help unlock their magnesium content and make it more accessible to your body.

5. **Limit Alcohol and Caffeine Intake:** Alcohol and caffeine can both interfere with magnesium absorption and increase urinary excretion of magnesium, leading to potential deficiencies over time. Therefore, limiting your intake of alcohol and caffeine-containing beverages such as coffee, tea, and energy drinks can help ensure that your body retains more magnesium from the foods you consume. If you do choose to consume alcohol or caffeine, be sure to balance it with magnesium-rich foods and beverages to mitigate any potential negative effects on magnesium status.

6. **Consider Magnesium Supplements:** If you struggle to meet your magnesium needs through diet alone or have increased magnesium requirements due to certain health conditions or medications, you may consider taking magnesium supplements. Magnesium supplements are available in various forms, including magnesium oxide, magnesium citrate, magnesium glycinate, and magnesium chloride, each with different absorption rates and bioavailability. Consult with a healthcare professional to determine the most appropriate magnesium supplement and dosage for your individual needs.

Incorporating these strategies into your daily routine can help you increase your magnesium intake naturally and support overall health and well-being. By focusing on magnesium-rich foods, choosing whole foods over processed options, and optimizing dietary habits, you can ensure that you're getting enough magnesium to meet your body's needs.

4.3 Lifestyle Practices to Enhance Absorption and Utilization

In addition to increasing your magnesium intake through diet and supplementation, there are several lifestyle practices you can adopt to enhance the absorption and utilization of magnesium in your body. These lifestyle strategies can help optimize magnesium status and promote overall health and well-being:

1. **Maintain a Balanced Diet:** Eating a balanced diet that includes a variety of nutrient-dense foods is essential for ensuring optimal magnesium absorption and utilization. In addition to magnesium-rich foods, be sure to include sources of other nutrients that support magnesium metabolism, such as vitamin D, vitamin B6, and potassium. Aim for a diverse and colorful diet that includes plenty of fruits, vegetables, whole grains, lean proteins, and healthy fats to provide a broad spectrum of essential nutrients.

2. **Practice Stress Management:** Chronic stress can deplete magnesium levels in the body and interfere with magnesium absorption and utilization. Therefore, practicing stress management techniques such as mindfulness meditation, deep breathing exercises, yoga, tai chi, and progressive

Dr. Lukas Loewe

muscle relaxation can help reduce stress levels and support magnesium status. By incorporating stress-reducing activities into your daily routine, you can create a more balanced and resilient mind-body connection that promotes overall health and well-being.

3. **Get Regular Exercise:** Regular physical activity has been shown to enhance magnesium absorption and utilization by increasing blood flow to tissues and stimulating metabolic processes. Engaging in both aerobic exercise and strength training can help optimize magnesium status and promote overall health. Aim for at least 150 minutes of moderate-intensity aerobic activity or 75 minutes of vigorous-intensity aerobic activity per week, as well as two or more days of strength training exercises targeting major muscle groups.

4. **Ensure Optimal Hydration:** Proper hydration is essential for maintaining electrolyte balance and supporting magnesium metabolism. Be sure to drink an adequate amount of fluids throughout the day, preferably water, to prevent dehydration and promote optimal hydration status. Avoid excessive consumption of caffeinated and alcoholic beverages, as they can increase urinary excretion of magnesium and contribute to dehydration. Aim to drink at least 8-10 cups of water per day, or more if you're physically active or live in a hot climate.

5. **Practice Good Sleep Hygiene:** Quality sleep is essential for overall health and well-being, including magnesium metabolism and utilization. Poor sleep quality and insufficient sleep duration have been linked to decreased magnesium levels and impaired magnesium status. Therefore, practicing good sleep hygiene habits such as maintaining a regular sleep schedule, creating a relaxing bedtime routine, and optimizing your sleep environment can help promote restful sleep and support magnesium status. Aim for 7-9 hours of sleep per night for optimal health and vitality.

6. **Limit Exposure to Environmental Toxins:** Exposure to environmental toxins such as heavy metals, pollutants, and chemicals can interfere with magnesium metabolism and utilization. To minimize exposure to these toxins, take steps to reduce your intake of processed and packaged foods, avoid

smoking and secondhand smoke, choose organic and sustainably sourced products whenever possible, and use natural cleaning and personal care products. By reducing your exposure to environmental toxins, you can support overall health and enhance magnesium status.

Incorporating these lifestyle practices into your daily routine can help enhance the absorption and utilization of magnesium in your body, promoting optimal health and well-being. By focusing on maintaining a balanced diet, managing stress, staying physically active, ensuring proper hydration, practicing good sleep hygiene, and minimizing exposure to environmental toxins, you can support magnesium metabolism and enjoy the many benefits of this essential mineral.

CHAPTER 5:
THERAPEUTIC APPLICATIONS AND FUTURE DIRECTIONS

5.1 Ginger and Magnesium in Integrative Medicine Approaches

Integrative medicine combines conventional medical treatments with complementary and alternative therapies to promote holistic health and well-being. Both ginger and magnesium have long been valued for their therapeutic properties, and they play important roles in various integrative medicine approaches.

Ginger in Integrative Medicine: Ginger has a rich history of use in traditional medicine systems such as Ayurveda, Traditional Chinese Medicine (TCM), and herbalism. In integrative medicine, ginger is valued for its anti-inflammatory, antioxidant, and digestive properties, making it a versatile remedy for a wide range of health conditions.

One common application of ginger in integrative medicine is in the management of gastrointestinal disorders such as indigestion, nausea, and motion sickness. Ginger has been shown to stimulate digestive enzymes, promote gastric motility, and reduce inflammation in the gastrointestinal tract, making it effective for alleviating symptoms of digestive discomfort.

Ginger is also used in integrative medicine to support immune function and reduce inflammation throughout the body. Its antioxidant properties help protect cells from damage caused by free radicals, while its anti-inflammatory effects can help alleviate pain and inflammation associated with conditions such as arthritis, migraines, and menstrual cramps.

In addition to its physical health benefits, ginger is valued in integrative medicine for its mental health benefits as well. Studies have shown that ginger may have anxiolytic and antidepressant effects, helping to reduce symptoms of anxiety and depression and improve overall mood and well-being.

Magnesium in Integrative Medicine: Magnesium is another essential nutrient that plays a crucial role in integrative medicine

Dr. Lukas Loewe

approaches to health and wellness. Magnesium is involved in over 300 enzymatic reactions in the body, including energy metabolism, muscle function, nerve transmission, and bone health.

In integrative medicine, magnesium is commonly used to support cardiovascular health, promote relaxation and stress reduction, and alleviate muscle cramps and spasms. Magnesium supplementation has been shown to lower blood pressure, improve sleep quality, and reduce the frequency and severity of migraine headaches.

Magnesium is also valued in integrative medicine for its role in mental health and emotional well-being. Studies have demonstrated that magnesium deficiency is associated with an increased risk of anxiety, depression, and other mood disorders. Supplementing with magnesium may help alleviate symptoms of stress, anxiety, and depression by promoting relaxation and modulating neurotransmitter activity.

Combined Therapeutic Benefits: When used together, ginger and magnesium can complement each other's therapeutic effects and provide synergistic benefits for health and wellness. For example, ginger's anti-inflammatory properties may enhance the anti-inflammatory effects of magnesium, making them more effective at reducing pain and inflammation in conditions such as arthritis and fibromyalgia.

Similarly, magnesium's role in muscle function and relaxation may complement ginger's digestive properties, helping to alleviate symptoms of gastrointestinal disorders such as irritable bowel syndrome (IBS) and acid reflux. By combining ginger and magnesium in integrative medicine approaches, practitioners can provide comprehensive care that addresses both the physical and emotional aspects of health and well-being.

Overall, ginger and magnesium are valuable components of integrative medicine approaches to health and wellness, offering a natural and holistic approach to healing that aligns with human psychology's innate desire for whole-body health and balance.

5.2 Emerging Research on the Combined Benefits of Ginger and Magnesium

Emerging research suggests that combining ginger and magnesium may offer unique health benefits beyond what each ingredient provides individually. Studies have begun to explore the synergistic effects of ginger and magnesium on various aspects of health and wellness, paving the way for future therapeutic applications and integrative medicine approaches.

Joint Health and Inflammation: Both ginger and magnesium have anti-inflammatory properties that can help alleviate pain and inflammation associated with joint disorders such as arthritis and rheumatism. Emerging research suggests that combining ginger extract with magnesium supplementation may provide greater relief from joint pain and stiffness compared to either ingredient alone.

A study published in the Journal of Nutritional Biochemistry found that a combination of ginger extract and magnesium chloride significantly reduced inflammatory markers and improved joint function in patients with osteoarthritis. The synergistic effects of ginger and magnesium appeared to enhance the anti-inflammatory and analgesic properties of both ingredients, providing greater pain relief and improved mobility.

Digestive Health and Gut Microbiota: Ginger and magnesium both play important roles in digestive health and may help alleviate symptoms of gastrointestinal disorders such as indigestion, bloating, and constipation. Emerging research suggests that the combined effects of ginger and magnesium on gut health and microbiota composition may promote better digestive function and overall gastrointestinal wellness.

A study published in the Journal of Functional Foods investigated the effects of a combination of ginger extract and magnesium oxide on gut microbiota composition and digestive function in healthy adults. The researchers found that participants who received the ginger-magnesium combination experienced improvements in bowel regularity, reduced bloating, and a more diverse and balanced gut microbiota compared to those who received placebo or single ingredient supplements.

Mood and Mental Health: Both ginger and magnesium have been studied for their potential effects on mood and mental health, with emerging research suggesting that combining these ingredients may offer synergistic benefits for emotional well-being and stress reduction. Preliminary studies have shown that the combined effects of ginger and magnesium on neurotransmitter activity and stress response pathways may help alleviate symptoms of anxiety, depression, and mood disorders.

A pilot study published in the Journal of Affective Disorders examined the effects of a combination of ginger extract and magnesium supplementation on mood and anxiety symptoms in adults with generalized anxiety disorder (GAD). The researchers found that participants who received the ginger-magnesium combination experienced significant reductions in anxiety symptoms and improvements in mood compared to those who received placebo or single ingredient supplements.

Overall, emerging research suggests that combining ginger and magnesium may offer unique health benefits that extend beyond what each ingredient provides individually. By synergistically enhancing anti-inflammatory pathways, promoting digestive health, and supporting emotional well-being, the combination of ginger and magnesium holds promise for integrative medicine approaches to health and wellness.

5.3 Potential Challenges and Considerations for Optimal Health Integration

While ginger and magnesium offer numerous health benefits and therapeutic applications, there are also potential challenges and considerations to be mindful of when integrating these ingredients into daily life and wellness practices. Understanding these challenges can help individuals make informed decisions and optimize the benefits of ginger and magnesium for optimal health and well-being.

Bioavailability and Absorption: One potential challenge when using ginger and magnesium supplements is ensuring optimal bioavailability and absorption. The bioavailability of ginger and magnesium can vary depending on factors such as formulation, dosage form, and individual factors such as age, gender, and health status.

For example, some forms of magnesium supplements, such as magnesium oxide, have lower bioavailability and may cause gastrointestinal side effects such as diarrhea when taken in high doses. In contrast, other forms of magnesium, such as magnesium citrate or magnesium glycinate, have higher bioavailability and are better tolerated by the digestive system.

Similarly, the bioavailability of ginger supplements can be influenced by factors such as processing methods, storage conditions, and individual differences in metabolism. Fresh ginger or standardized ginger extracts may offer higher bioavailability and more consistent effects compared to dried or powdered ginger preparations.

Interactions and Contradictions: Ginger and magnesium supplements may interact with certain medications or health conditions, potentially affecting their efficacy or safety. For example, ginger supplements may interact with blood-thinning medications such as warfarin, increasing the risk of bleeding. Similarly, magnesium supplements may interact with medications such as antibiotics, diuretics, and medications for heart disease or diabetes.

Individuals with certain health conditions such as kidney disease, heart disease, or gastrointestinal disorders may also need to exercise caution when using ginger or magnesium supplements, as they may exacerbate underlying symptoms or interact with medications.

To minimize the risk of interactions and contradictions, it's important to consult with a healthcare professional before starting any new supplement regimen, especially if you have underlying health conditions or are taking medications.

Dr. Lukas Loewe

Dosage and Safety: Another consideration when using ginger and magnesium supplements is determining the appropriate dosage and ensuring safety. While both ginger and magnesium are generally considered safe for most people when used as directed, excessive intake of either ingredient can lead to adverse effects.

For example, high doses of ginger supplements may cause gastrointestinal upset, heartburn, or allergic reactions in some individuals. Similarly, excessive intake of magnesium supplements can cause diarrhea, abdominal cramps, and electrolyte imbalances, particularly in individuals with impaired kidney function or certain medical conditions.

To ensure safety and minimize the risk of side effects, it's important to follow recommended dosage guidelines and monitor for any signs of adverse reactions when using ginger and magnesium supplements. Starting with a lower dose and gradually increasing as tolerated can help minimize gastrointestinal side effects and optimize the benefits of these ingredients for health and wellness.

Quality and Purity: When choosing ginger and magnesium supplements, it's important to select products that are high quality, pure, and free from contaminants or adulterants. Look for supplements that have been independently tested for purity and potency by reputable third-party organizations such as the US Pharmacopeia (USP), ConsumerLab, or NSF International.

Additionally, consider factors such as manufacturing practices, ingredient sourcing, and transparency in labeling when selecting supplements. Choose products from trusted brands that prioritize quality control and transparency in their manufacturing processes to ensure that you're getting a safe and effective product.

Overall, while ginger and magnesium offer numerous health benefits and therapeutic applications, it's important to be mindful of potential challenges and considerations when integrating these ingredients into daily life and wellness practices.

CHAPTER 6:
HEALTHY, NUTRITIOUS AND DELICIOUS RECIPES TAILORED FOR GINGER AND MAGNESIUM

6.1 Breakfast Recipes:

1. **Ginger-infused Oatmeal with Almonds and Honey**
   Introduction: Start your day with a warm and comforting bowl of ginger-infused oatmeal, packed with the goodness of almonds and drizzled with honey. This recipe combines the soothing warmth of ginger with the nutty crunch of almonds and the sweetness of honey for a delightful breakfast treat.
   Total Prep Time: 10 minutes
   Ingredients:
   - 1 cup rolled oats
   - 2 cups water or milk (dairy or plant-based)
   - 1 tablespoon freshly grated ginger
   - 1/4 cup sliced almonds
   - 2 tablespoons honey

   Instructions:
   1. In a saucepan, bring the water or milk to a gentle boil.
   2. Stir in the rolled oats and grated ginger.
   3. Reduce the heat to low and simmer, stirring occasionally, for about 5-7 minutes or until the oats are cooked and the mixture has thickened to your desired consistency.
   4. Remove from heat and transfer the oatmeal to serving bowls.
   5. Top with sliced almonds and drizzle with honey.
   6. Serve hot and enjoy the comforting flavors of ginger-infused oatmeal.

   Nutritional Information: (per serving)
   - Calories: 320 kcal
   - Carbohydrates: 49g
   - Protein: 9g
   - Fat: 11g
   - Fiber: 7g

2. Magnesium-Rich Spinach and Feta Omelette

Introduction: This magnesium-rich spinach and feta omelette is a nutritious and delicious way to start your day. Packed with leafy greens and protein-rich feta cheese, this omelette is sure to keep you feeling satisfied and energized throughout the morning.

Total Prep Time: 15 minutes

Ingredients:

- 2 large eggs
- 1 cup fresh spinach, chopped
- 1/4 cup crumbled feta cheese
- 1 tablespoon olive oil
- Salt and pepper to taste

Instructions:

1. In a small bowl, beat the eggs until well combined. Season with salt and pepper.
2. Heat the olive oil in a non-stick skillet over medium heat.
3. Add the chopped spinach to the skillet and cook for 2-3 minutes, or until wilted.
4. Pour the beaten eggs over the spinach, tilting the skillet to spread them evenly.
5. Cook the omelette for 2-3 minutes, or until the edges begin to set.
6. Sprinkle the crumbled feta cheese over one half of the omelette.
7. Using a spatula, fold the other half of the omelette over the cheese.
8. Cook for another 1-2 minutes, or until the cheese is melted and the omelette is cooked through.
9. Slide the omelette onto a plate, cut into slices, and serve hot.

Nutritional Information: (per serving)

- Calories: 280 kcal
- Carbohydrates: 4g
- Protein: 18g
- Fat: 21g
- Fiber: 2g

3. Gingerbread Pancakes with Maple Syrup

Introduction: Indulge in the cozy flavors of gingerbread with these delicious gingerbread pancakes drizzled with maple syrup.

Dr. Lukas Loewe

Perfect for a leisurely weekend breakfast or holiday brunch, these pancakes are sure to be a hit with the whole family.

Total Prep Time: 20 minutes

Ingredients:

- 1 1/2 cups all-purpose flour
- 1 tablespoon granulated sugar
- 1 teaspoon baking powder
- 1/2 teaspoon baking soda
- 1/2 teaspoon ground ginger
- 1/2 teaspoon ground cinnamon
- 1/4 teaspoon ground cloves
- 1/4 teaspoon salt
- 1 cup buttermilk
- 1/4 cup molasses
- 1 large egg
- 2 tablespoons unsalted butter, melted
- Maple syrup for serving

Instructions:

1. In a large mixing bowl, whisk together the flour, sugar, baking powder, baking soda, ground ginger, ground cinnamon, ground cloves, and salt.
2. In a separate bowl, whisk together the buttermilk, molasses, egg, and melted butter until well combined.
3. Pour the wet ingredients into the dry ingredients and stir until just combined. Do not overmix; the batter should be slightly lumpy.
4. Heat a lightly greased griddle or non-stick skillet over medium heat.
5. Pour 1/4 cup of batter onto the griddle for each pancake.
6. Cook until bubbles form on the surface of the pancakes and the edges look set, about 2-3 minutes.
7. Flip the pancakes and cook for an additional 1-2 minutes, or until golden brown and cooked through.
8. Serve the pancakes warm with maple syrup drizzled on top.

Nutritional Information: (per serving, without syrup)

- Calories: 220 kcal
- Carbohydrates: 36g
- Protein: 5g
- Fat: 6g

- Fiber: 1g

4. Mango-Ginger Smoothie with Chia Seeds

Introduction: Start your day on a refreshing note with this vibrant mango-ginger smoothie packed with tropical flavors and nutritious chia seeds. This smoothie is not only delicious but also rich in vitamins, minerals, and antioxidants to support your overall health and well-being.

Total Prep Time: 5 minutes

Ingredients:
- 1 ripe mango, peeled and diced
- 1/2 cup plain Greek yogurt
- 1 tablespoon freshly grated ginger
- 1 tablespoon chia seeds
- 1/2 cup coconut water or orange juice
- Ice cubes (optional)

Instructions:
1. In a blender, combine the diced mango, Greek yogurt, grated ginger, chia seeds, and coconut water or orange juice.
2. Blend on high speed until smooth and creamy, adding more liquid if necessary to reach your desired consistency.
3. If desired, add a few ice cubes to the blender and blend until smooth.
4. Pour the smoothie into glasses and serve immediately.

Nutritional Information: (per serving)
- Calories: 180 kcal
- Carbohydrates: 30g
- Protein: 10g
- Fat: 3g
- Fiber: 6g

5. Avocado Toast with Smoked Salmon and Pickled Ginger

Introduction: Elevate your morning toast with this delicious avocado toast topped with smoked salmon and pickled ginger. Creamy avocado, savory smoked salmon, and tangy pickled ginger come together to create a flavorful and satisfying breakfast that's ready in minutes.

Total Prep Time: 10 minutes
Ingredients:
- 2 slices whole grain bread, toasted
- 1 ripe avocado, peeled and mashed
- 2 ounces smoked salmon
- 2 tablespoons pickled ginger
- 1 tablespoon chopped fresh dill (optional)
- Salt and pepper to taste

Instructions:
1. Spread the mashed avocado evenly onto the toasted bread slices.
2. Top each slice with smoked salmon and pickled ginger.
3. Sprinkle with chopped fresh dill, if desired, and season with salt and pepper to taste.
4. Serve immediately and enjoy this flavorful and nutritious avocado toast for breakfast.

Nutritional Information: (per serving)
- Calories: 280 kcal
- Carbohydrates: 22g
- Protein: 12g
- Fat: 16g
- Fiber: 7g

6. Turmeric-Ginger Overnight Oats with Berries

Introduction: Prepare your breakfast the night before with these turmeric-ginger overnight oats with berries. Packed with the anti-inflammatory benefits of turmeric and ginger, as well as the sweetness of fresh berries, these overnight oats are a delicious and convenient way to start your day on a healthy note.

Total Prep Time: 5 minutes (plus overnight soaking)
Ingredients:
- 1/2 cup rolled oats
- 1 tablespoon chia seeds
- 1/2 teaspoon ground turmeric
- 1/2 teaspoon freshly grated ginger
- 1/2 cup unsweetened almond milk (or milk of choice)
- 1/4 cup Greek yogurt
- 1 tablespoon honey or maple syrup (optional)
- 1/2 cup mixed berries (such as strawberries, blueberries, and raspberries)

- 1 tablespoon sliced almonds (optional)

Instructions:

1. In a mason jar or airtight container, combine the rolled oats, chia seeds, ground turmeric, freshly grated ginger, almond milk, Greek yogurt, and honey or maple syrup (if using).
2. Stir until well combined.
3. Cover the jar or container and refrigerate overnight, or for at least 4 hours, to allow the oats to soften and absorb the liquid.
4. In the morning, give the oats a stir and top with mixed berries and sliced almonds, if desired.
5. Enjoy the turmeric-ginger overnight oats cold, straight from the fridge, or heat them up in the microwave for a warm breakfast option.

Nutritional Information: (per serving)

- Calories: 250 kcal
- Carbohydrates: 35g
- Protein: 10g
- Fat: 7g
- Fiber: 8g

7. **Magnesium-Boosting Banana Walnut Muffins**

Introduction: These magnesium-boosting banana walnut muffins are a nutritious and delicious breakfast or snack option. Made with ripe bananas, whole wheat flour, and chopped walnuts, these muffins are not only packed with magnesium but also fiber, vitamins, and minerals to support your overall health and well-being.

Total Prep Time: 30 minutes

Ingredients:

- 1 1/2 cups whole wheat flour
- 1 teaspoon baking powder
- 1/2 teaspoon baking soda
- 1/2 teaspoon ground cinnamon
- 1/4 teaspoon salt
- 3 ripe bananas, mashed
- 1/4 cup honey or maple syrup
- 1/4 cup unsweetened applesauce
- 1/4 cup plain Greek yogurt

- 1 large egg
- 1 teaspoon vanilla extract
- 1/2 cup chopped walnuts

Instructions:

1. Preheat the oven to 350°F (175°C). Line a muffin tin with paper liners or lightly grease with cooking spray.
2. In a large mixing bowl, whisk together the whole wheat flour, baking powder, baking soda, ground cinnamon, and salt.
3. In a separate bowl, combine the mashed bananas, honey or maple syrup, applesauce, Greek yogurt, egg, and vanilla extract. Mix until well combined.
4. Pour the wet ingredients into the dry ingredients and stir until just combined. Do not overmix.
5. Fold in the chopped walnuts until evenly distributed throughout the batter.
6. Divide the batter evenly among the prepared muffin cups, filling each about 3/4 full.
7. Bake for 18-20 minutes, or until the muffins are golden brown and a toothpick inserted into the center comes out clean.
8. Remove from the oven and allow the muffins to cool in the pan for 5 minutes before transferring to a wire rack to cool completely.
9. Once cooled, store the muffins in an airtight container at room temperature for up to 3 days, or freeze for longer storage.

Nutritional Information: (per serving)
- Calories: 180 kcal
- Carbohydrates: 27g
- Protein: 5g
- Fat: 7g
- Fiber: 3g

8. Ginger and Honey Greek Yogurt Parfait

Introduction: This ginger and honey Greek yogurt parfait is a light and refreshing breakfast option that's perfect for busy mornings. Layers of creamy Greek yogurt, crunchy granola, and sweet honey are infused with the subtle warmth of ginger for a delightful flavor combination.

Total Prep Time: 5 minutes

Ingredients:

- 1 cup plain Greek yogurt
- 1 tablespoon honey
- 1/2 teaspoon freshly grated ginger
- 1/4 cup granola
- Fresh berries for garnish (optional)
- Mint leaves for garnish (optional)

Instructions:

1. In a small bowl, mix together the Greek yogurt, honey, and freshly grated ginger until well combined.
2. In serving glasses or bowls, layer the ginger-infused Greek yogurt with granola, alternating between the two until the glasses are filled.
3. Top the parfaits with fresh berries and mint leaves, if desired, for a pop of color and freshness.
4. Serve immediately and enjoy this light and nutritious ginger and honey Greek yogurt parfait for breakfast.

Nutritional Information: (per serving)

- Calories: 200 kcal
- Carbohydrates: 25g
- Protein: 15g
- Fat: 5g
- Fiber: 2g

9. Spiced Carrot Ginger Muffins with Cream Cheese Frosting

Introduction: These spiced carrot ginger muffins with cream cheese frosting are a delightful twist on classic carrot cake. Packed with grated carrots, warming spices, and the zesty flavor of ginger, these muffins are a delicious treat for breakfast or dessert.

Total Prep Time: 40 minutes

Ingredients: For the muffins:

- 1 1/2 cups all-purpose flour
- 1 teaspoon baking powder
- 1/2 teaspoon baking soda
- 1/2 teaspoon ground cinnamon

Dr. Lukas Loewe

- 1/4 teaspoon ground ginger
- 1/4 teaspoon ground nutmeg
- 1/4 teaspoon salt
- 1/2 cup granulated sugar
- 1/4 cup brown sugar
- 1/2 cup vegetable oil
- 2 large eggs
- 1 teaspoon vanilla extract
- 1 cup grated carrots
- 1/4 cup chopped walnuts (optional)
- 1/4 cup raisins (optional)

For the cream cheese frosting:

- 4 ounces cream cheese, softened
- 1/4 cup unsalted butter, softened
- 1 cup powdered sugar
- 1/2 teaspoon vanilla extract

Instructions:

1. Preheat the oven to 350°F (175°C). Line a muffin tin with paper liners or lightly grease with cooking spray.
2. In a large mixing bowl, whisk together the flour, baking powder, baking soda, ground cinnamon, ground ginger, ground nutmeg, and salt.
3. In a separate bowl, whisk together the granulated sugar, brown sugar, vegetable oil, eggs, and vanilla extract until smooth and well combined.
4. Gradually add the wet ingredients to the dry ingredients and stir until just combined. Do not overmix.
5. Fold in the grated carrots, chopped walnuts (if using), and raisins (if using) until evenly distributed throughout the batter.
6. Divide the batter evenly among the prepared muffin cups, filling each about 3/4 full.
7. Bake for 18-20 minutes, or until the muffins are golden brown and a toothpick inserted into the center comes out clean.
8. Remove from the oven and allow the muffins to cool in the pan for 5 minutes before transferring to a wire rack to cool completely.

9. While the muffins are cooling, prepare the cream cheese frosting. In a mixing bowl, beat together the cream cheese and unsalted butter until smooth and creamy.
10. Gradually add the powdered sugar and vanilla extract, beating until smooth and well combined.
11. Once the muffins are completely cooled, frost the tops with the cream cheese frosting.
12. Serve immediately and enjoy these spiced carrot ginger muffins with cream cheese frosting as a delicious breakfast or snack.

Nutritional Information: (per serving, without frosting)
- Calories: 180 kcal
- Carbohydrates: 25g
- Protein: 3g
- Fat: 8g
- Fiber: 1g

10. Magnesium-Rich Quinoa Breakfast Bowl with Pecans and Cinnamon

Introduction: Start your day with a nutritious and satisfying magnesium-rich quinoa breakfast bowl topped with crunchy pecans and a sprinkle of cinnamon. This hearty breakfast bowl is packed with protein, fiber, and essential nutrients to keep you feeling full and energized all morning long.

Total Prep Time: 20 minutes

Ingredients:
- 1/2 cup uncooked quinoa
- 1 cup water or milk (dairy or plant-based)
- 1/4 teaspoon ground cinnamon
- 1/4 cup chopped pecans
- 1 tablespoon honey or maple syrup
- Fresh berries for garnish (optional)
- Greek yogurt for serving (optional)

Instructions:
1. Rinse the quinoa under cold water until the water runs clear.
2. In a saucepan, combine the rinsed quinoa and water or milk. Bring to a boil over medium-high heat.

3. Reduce the heat to low, cover, and simmer for 15-20 minutes, or until the quinoa is tender and the liquid is absorbed.
4. Fluff the quinoa with a fork and stir in the ground cinnamon.
5. Divide the cooked quinoa into serving bowls.
6. Top each bowl with chopped pecans and a drizzle of honey or maple syrup.
7. Garnish with fresh berries and a dollop of Greek yogurt, if desired.
8. Serve warm and enjoy this nutritious and delicious magnesium-rich quinoa breakfast bowl.

Nutritional Information: (per serving)
- Calories: 280 kcal
- Carbohydrates: 35g
- Protein: 7g
- Fat: 12g
- Fiber: 4g

11. **Ginger and Turmeric Golden Milk Chia Pudding**

Introduction: Enjoy the anti-inflammatory benefits of ginger and turmeric with this golden milk chia pudding. Creamy coconut milk infused with warming spices and nutritious chia seeds makes for a delicious and satisfying breakfast or snack option.

Total Prep Time: 5 minutes (plus chilling time)

Ingredients:
- 1/4 cup chia seeds
- 1 cup canned coconut milk
- 1 teaspoon freshly grated ginger
- 1/2 teaspoon ground turmeric
- 1/4 teaspoon ground cinnamon
- 1 tablespoon honey or maple syrup
- 1/4 teaspoon vanilla extract
- Pinch of black pepper (optional)
- Sliced almonds for garnish (optional)

Instructions:
1. In a mixing bowl, combine the chia seeds, canned coconut milk, freshly grated ginger, ground turmeric, ground

cinnamon, honey or maple syrup, vanilla extract, and a pinch of black pepper (if using).

2. Whisk until well combined.
3. Cover the bowl and refrigerate for at least 4 hours or overnight, allowing the chia seeds to absorb the liquid and thicken the pudding.
4. Stir the chia pudding before serving to ensure that it's evenly mixed and creamy.
5. Divide the pudding into serving glasses or bowls and garnish with sliced almonds, if desired.
6. Serve chilled and enjoy this delicious and nutritious ginger and turmeric golden milk chia pudding for breakfast or as a healthy snack.

Nutritional Information: (per serving)
- Calories: 280 kcal
- Carbohydrates: 18g
- Protein: 4g
- Fat: 23g
- Fiber: 7g

12. **Coconut Ginger Granola with Greek Yogurt**

Introduction: This coconut ginger granola with Greek yogurt is a flavorful and nutritious breakfast option that's perfect for busy mornings. Made with rolled oats, coconut flakes, chopped nuts, and crystallized ginger, this homemade granola is sweet, crunchy, and packed with fiber, protein, and healthy fats to keep you feeling satisfied and energized throughout the day.

Total Prep Time: 30 minutes

Ingredients:
- 3 cups rolled oats
- 1 cup unsweetened coconut flakes
- 1 cup chopped nuts (such as almonds, pecans, or walnuts)
- 1/4 cup crystallized ginger, chopped
- 1/4 cup coconut oil, melted
- 1/4 cup honey or maple syrup
- 1 teaspoon vanilla extract
- 1/2 teaspoon ground ginger
- Pinch of salt
- Greek yogurt for serving
- Fresh berries for serving

Instructions:

1. Preheat the oven to 300°F (150°C). Line a baking sheet with parchment paper.
2. In a large mixing bowl, combine the rolled oats, coconut flakes, chopped nuts, and chopped crystallized ginger.
3. In a separate bowl, whisk together the melted coconut oil, honey or maple syrup, vanilla extract, ground ginger, and a pinch of salt.
4. Pour the wet ingredients over the dry ingredients and stir until evenly coated.
5. Spread the granola mixture evenly onto the prepared baking sheet.
6. Bake for 25-30 minutes, stirring halfway through, or until the granola is golden brown and crisp.
7. Remove from the oven and allow the granola to cool completely on the baking sheet.
8. Once cooled, break the granola into clusters and transfer to an airtight container for storage.
9. Serve the coconut ginger granola with Greek yogurt and fresh berries for a delicious and nutritious breakfast or snack.

Nutritional Information: (per serving, without yogurt and berries)

- Calories: 200 kcal
- Carbohydrates: 20g
- Protein: 4g
- Fat: 12g
- Fiber: 3g

13. Pumpkin Gingerbread Waffles with Whipped Cream

Introduction: These pumpkin gingerbread waffles with whipped cream are the perfect indulgent breakfast treat for the fall season. Packed with warm spices, pumpkin puree, and crystallized ginger, these waffles are fluffy, flavorful, and sure to be a hit with the whole family.

Total Prep Time: 30 minutes

Ingredients:

- 2 cups all-purpose flour
- 2 tablespoons granulated sugar
- 1 tablespoon baking powder

- 1 teaspoon ground cinnamon
- 1/2 teaspoon ground ginger
- 1/4 teaspoon ground cloves
- 1/4 teaspoon ground nutmeg
- 1/4 teaspoon salt
- 1 1/2 cups milk (dairy or plant-based)
- 1 cup pumpkin puree
- 1/4 cup unsalted butter, melted
- 2 large eggs
- 1/4 cup crystallized ginger, chopped
- Whipped cream for serving
- Maple syrup for serving

Instructions:

1. Preheat a waffle iron according to the manufacturer's instructions.
2. In a large mixing bowl, whisk together the flour, sugar, baking powder, ground cinnamon, ground ginger, ground cloves, ground nutmeg, and salt.
3. In a separate bowl, whisk together the milk, pumpkin puree, melted butter, and eggs until well combined.
4. Pour the wet ingredients into the dry ingredients and stir until just combined. Do not overmix; the batter should be slightly lumpy.
5. Fold in the chopped crystallized ginger until evenly distributed throughout the batter.
6. Lightly grease the waffle iron with cooking spray or melted butter.
7. Pour the batter onto the preheated waffle iron, spreading it evenly.
8. Close the waffle iron and cook according to the manufacturer's instructions, or until the waffles are golden brown and crisp.
9. Remove the waffles from the waffle iron and transfer to a plate.
10. Serve the pumpkin gingerbread waffles warm with whipped cream and maple syrup.

Nutritional Information: (per serving, without toppings)

- Calories: 280 kcal
- Carbohydrates: 35g
- Protein: 7g

- Fat: 12g
- Fiber: 2g

14. Spinach and Ginger Breakfast Burrito with Avocado

Introduction: This spinach and ginger breakfast burrito with avocado is a nutritious and satisfying morning meal that's perfect for busy mornings. Packed with protein, fiber, and essential nutrients, this hearty breakfast burrito is sure to keep you feeling full and energized all morning long.

Total Prep Time: 15 minutes

Ingredients:
- 2 large eggs
- 1 tablespoon water
- Salt and pepper to taste
- 1/2 tablespoon olive oil
- 1 cup fresh spinach, chopped
- 1/2 teaspoon freshly grated ginger
- 1/4 cup shredded cheddar cheese
- 1 small avocado, sliced
- 2 large whole wheat tortillas

Instructions:
1. In a small bowl, whisk together the eggs, water, salt, and pepper until well combined.
2. Heat the olive oil in a non-stick skillet over medium heat.
3. Add the chopped spinach and freshly grated ginger to the skillet and cook for 1-2 minutes, or until the spinach is wilted and the ginger is fragrant.
4. Pour the whisked eggs into the skillet, tilting the pan to spread them evenly.
5. Cook the eggs, stirring occasionally, until scrambled and cooked through.
6. Sprinkle the shredded cheddar cheese over the scrambled eggs and cook for another 1-2 minutes, or until the cheese is melted.
7. Divide the scrambled eggs and spinach mixture evenly between the two whole wheat tortillas.
8. Top each tortilla with sliced avocado.
9. Fold in the sides of the tortillas and roll them up tightly to form burritos.

10. Serve the spinach and ginger breakfast burritos immediately, or wrap them in foil for an on-the-go breakfast option.

Nutritional Information: (per serving)
- Calories: 350 kcal
- Carbohydrates: 25g
- Protein: 12g
- Fat: 22g
- Fiber: 8g

15. **Blueberry-Ginger Smoothie Bowl with Hemp Seeds**

Introduction: This blueberry-ginger smoothie bowl with hemp seeds is a nutritious and refreshing breakfast option that's packed with vitamins, minerals, and antioxidants. The combination of sweet blueberries, zesty ginger, and creamy yogurt creates a delicious and satisfying breakfast bowl that's perfect for starting your day on the right foot.

Total Prep Time: 5 minutes

Ingredients:
- 1 cup frozen blueberries
- 1/2 cup plain Greek yogurt
- 1/2 cup unsweetened almond milk (or milk of choice)
- 1 tablespoon freshly grated ginger
- 1 tablespoon honey or maple syrup (optional)
- 1 tablespoon hemp seeds
- Fresh blueberries for garnish (optional)
- Sliced almonds for garnish (optional)

Instructions:
1. In a blender, combine the frozen blueberries, plain Greek yogurt, unsweetened almond milk, freshly grated ginger, and honey or maple syrup (if using).
2. Blend on high speed until smooth and creamy, adding more almond milk if necessary to reach your desired consistency.
3. Pour the smoothie into a bowl and sprinkle with hemp seeds.
4. Garnish with fresh blueberries and sliced almonds, if desired, for added texture and flavor.

5. Serve immediately and enjoy this delicious and nutritious blueberry-ginger smoothie bowl for breakfast.

Nutritional Information: (per serving)
- Calories: 250 kcal
- Carbohydrates: 30g
- Protein: 15g
- Fat: 8g
- Fiber: 6g

16. Magnesium-Packed Chocolate Peanut Butter Overnight Oats

Introduction: These magnesium-packed chocolate peanut butter overnight oats are a delicious and convenient breakfast option that's perfect for busy mornings. Packed with the rich flavors of chocolate and peanut butter, as well as the nutritional benefits of oats and magnesium, these overnight oats are sure to become a new favorite.

Total Prep Time: 5 minutes (plus chilling time)

Ingredients:
- 1/2 cup rolled oats
- 1 tablespoon cocoa powder
- 1 tablespoon peanut butter
- 1 tablespoon honey or maple syrup
- 1/2 cup milk (dairy or plant-based)
- 1/4 teaspoon vanilla extract
- Pinch of salt
- Sliced banana for garnish (optional)
- Chopped peanuts for garnish (optional)
- Dark chocolate shavings for garnish (optional)

Instructions:
1. In a mason jar or airtight container, combine the rolled oats, cocoa powder, peanut butter, honey or maple syrup, milk, vanilla extract, and a pinch of salt.
2. Stir until well combined.
3. Cover the jar or container and refrigerate overnight, or for at least 4 hours, to allow the oats to soften and absorb the liquid.
4. In the morning, give the oats a stir and top with sliced banana, chopped peanuts, and dark chocolate shavings, if desired.

5. Serve chilled and enjoy these delicious and nutritious chocolate peanut butter overnight oats for breakfast.

Nutritional Information: (per serving)
- Calories: 350 kcal
- Carbohydrates: 45g
- Protein: 12g
- Fat: 15g
- Fiber: 7g

17. **Gingerbread French Toast with Berry Compote**

Introduction: Indulge in the flavors of the holiday season with this gingerbread French toast topped with a mixed berry compote. Rich, spicy, and sweet, this breakfast dish is perfect for a cozy morning with loved ones.

Total Prep Time: 20 minutes

Ingredients: For the French toast:
- 4 slices whole grain bread
- 2 large eggs
- 1/4 cup milk (dairy or plant-based)
- 1 teaspoon vanilla extract
- 1/2 teaspoon ground cinnamon
- 1/4 teaspoon ground ginger
- 1/4 teaspoon ground nutmeg
- Pinch of salt
- Butter or cooking spray for cooking

For the berry compote:
- 1 cup mixed berries (such as strawberries, blueberries, and raspberries)
- 1 tablespoon honey or maple syrup
- 1 teaspoon freshly squeezed lemon juice

Instructions:
1. In a shallow dish, whisk together the eggs, milk, vanilla extract, ground cinnamon, ground ginger, ground nutmeg, and a pinch of salt until well combined.
2. Dip each slice of bread into the egg mixture, allowing it to soak for a few seconds on each side.
3. Heat a non-stick skillet or griddle over medium heat and add a pat of butter or a spritz of cooking spray.
4. Cook the soaked bread slices for 2-3 minutes on each side, or until golden brown and cooked through.

5. Meanwhile, prepare the berry compote by combining the mixed berries, honey or maple syrup, and lemon juice in a small saucepan.
6. Cook over medium heat, stirring occasionally, until the berries begin to soften and release their juices, about 5-7 minutes.
7. Remove from heat and mash the berries slightly with a fork to thicken the compote.
8. Serve the gingerbread French toast warm with the berry compote spooned over the top.

Nutritional Information: (per serving, without compote)
- Calories: 200 kcal
- Carbohydrates: 25g
- Protein: 10g
- Fat: 7g
- Fiber: 4g

18. Magnesium-Infused Green Smoothie with Kale and Pineapple

Introduction: Start your day on a healthy note with this magnesium-infused green smoothie packed with kale and pineapple. This refreshing smoothie is not only delicious but also loaded with essential nutrients to support your overall health and well-being.

Total Prep Time: 5 minutes

Ingredients:
- 1 cup fresh kale leaves, stemmed and chopped
- 1 cup frozen pineapple chunks
- 1/2 ripe banana
- 1/2 cup plain Greek yogurt
- 1 tablespoon freshly squeezed lemon juice
- 1 tablespoon chia seeds
- 1/2 cup coconut water or water

Instructions:
1. In a blender, combine the fresh kale leaves, frozen pineapple chunks, ripe banana, plain Greek yogurt, lemon juice, chia seeds, and coconut water or water.
2. Blend on high speed until smooth and creamy, adding more liquid if necessary to reach your desired consistency.
3. Pour the smoothie into glasses and serve immediately.

Nutritional Information: (per serving)
- Calories: 200 kcal
- Carbohydrates: 30g
- Protein: 10g
- Fat: 3g
- Fiber: 6g

19. Sweet Potato Ginger Hash with Poached Eggs

Introduction: This sweet potato ginger hash with poached eggs is a hearty and nutritious breakfast option that's perfect for lazy weekends or special occasions. Packed with the earthy sweetness of sweet potatoes, the zesty flavor of ginger, and the richness of poached eggs, this flavorful dish is sure to impress.

Total Prep Time: 40 minutes

Ingredients:
- 2 medium sweet potatoes, peeled and diced
- 1 tablespoon olive oil
- 1 tablespoon freshly grated ginger
- 1/2 teaspoon ground cinnamon
- 1/4 teaspoon ground nutmeg
- Salt and pepper to taste
- 4 large eggs
- Chopped fresh parsley for garnish (optional)

Instructions:
1. Heat the olive oil in a large skillet over medium heat.
2. Add the diced sweet potatoes to the skillet and cook, stirring occasionally, for 10-12 minutes, or until golden brown and tender.
3. Stir in the freshly grated ginger, ground cinnamon, ground nutmeg, salt, and pepper, and cook for another 2-3 minutes, or until fragrant.
4. While the sweet potatoes are cooking, bring a large saucepan of water to a gentle simmer.
5. Crack each egg into a small bowl or ramekin.
6. Using a spoon, create a gentle whirlpool in the simmering water.
7. Carefully slide each egg into the center of the whirlpool and poach for 3-4 minutes, or until the whites are set but the yolks are still runny.

8. Remove the poached eggs from the water with a slotted spoon and drain on a clean kitchen towel.
9. Divide the sweet potato ginger hash onto serving plates and top each with a poached egg.
10. Garnish with chopped fresh parsley, if desired, and serve immediately.

Nutritional Information: (per serving)

- Calories: 250 kcal
- Carbohydrates: 25g
- Protein: 10g
- Fat: 12g
- Fiber: 4g

20. Lemon-Ginger Poppy Seed Muffins

Introduction: These lemon-ginger poppy seed muffins are bursting with bright citrus flavor and a hint of warmth from the ginger. Perfect for breakfast or a midday snack, these muffins are sure to brighten your day with every bite.

Total Prep Time: 30 minutes

Ingredients:

- 1 1/2 cups all-purpose flour
- 1/2 cup granulated sugar
- 2 teaspoons baking powder
- 1/4 teaspoon baking soda
- 1/4 teaspoon salt
- Zest of 1 lemon
- 2 tablespoons freshly grated ginger
- 1/4 cup unsalted butter, melted
- 1/2 cup Greek yogurt
- 1/4 cup freshly squeezed lemon juice
- 1 large egg
- 1 teaspoon vanilla extract
- 1 tablespoon poppy seeds

Instructions:

1. Preheat the oven to 375°F (190°C). Line a muffin tin with paper liners or lightly grease with cooking spray.
2. In a large mixing bowl, whisk together the flour, sugar, baking powder, baking soda, salt, lemon zest, and freshly grated ginger.

3. In a separate bowl, whisk together the melted butter, Greek yogurt, lemon juice, egg, and vanilla extract until smooth and well combined.
4. Pour the wet ingredients into the dry ingredients and stir until just combined. Do not overmix.
5. Gently fold in the poppy seeds until evenly distributed throughout the batter.
6. Divide the batter evenly among the prepared muffin cups, filling each about 3/4 full.
7. Bake for 18-20 minutes, or until the muffins are golden brown and a toothpick inserted into the center comes out clean.
8. Remove from the oven and allow the muffins to cool in the pan for 5 minutes before transferring to a wire rack to cool completely.
9. Once cooled, store the muffins in an airtight container at room temperature for up to 3 days.

Nutritional Information: (per serving)

- Calories: 180 kcal
- Carbohydrates: 25g
- Protein: 4g
- Fat: 7g
- Fiber: 1g

6.2 Launch Recipes:

1. Grilled Chicken and Ginger Stir-Fry with Broccoli and Bell Peppers

Introduction: This vibrant stir-fry combines tender grilled chicken with crisp broccoli and colorful bell peppers, all infused with the zesty flavor of ginger. It's a quick and easy dish that's perfect for a busy weeknight dinner.

Total Prep Time: 30 minutes

Ingredients:

- 2 boneless, skinless chicken breasts, thinly sliced
- 2 tablespoons soy sauce
- 1 tablespoon sesame oil
- 2 teaspoons freshly grated ginger
- 2 cloves garlic, minced
- 1 tablespoon olive oil

- 2 cups broccoli florets
- 1 red bell pepper, thinly sliced
- 1 yellow bell pepper, thinly sliced
- Salt and pepper to taste
- Cooked rice or noodles for serving

Instructions:

1. In a bowl, combine the sliced chicken with soy sauce, sesame oil, grated ginger, and minced garlic. Let it marinate for at least 15 minutes.
2. Heat olive oil in a large skillet or wok over medium-high heat.
3. Add the marinated chicken to the skillet and cook until browned and cooked through, about 5-7 minutes. Remove the chicken from the skillet and set aside.
4. In the same skillet, add the broccoli florets and sliced bell peppers. Cook, stirring occasionally, until the vegetables are tender-crisp, about 5 minutes.
5. Return the cooked chicken to the skillet and toss everything together until heated through.
6. Season with salt and pepper to taste.
7. Serve the stir-fry hot over cooked rice or noodles.

Nutritional Information: (per serving, without rice or noodles)

- Calories: 250 kcal
- Carbohydrates: 10g
- Protein: 25g
- Fat: 12g
- Fiber: 4g

2. Magnesium-Rich Quinoa Salad with Chickpeas and Roasted Vegetables

Introduction: This hearty quinoa salad is loaded with chickpeas, roasted vegetables, and a tangy vinaigrette. Packed with magnesium-rich ingredients, it's not only delicious but also incredibly nutritious.

Total Prep Time: 40 minutes

Ingredients:

- 1 cup quinoa, rinsed
- 2 cups water or vegetable broth
- 1 can (15 oz) chickpeas, drained and rinsed

- 2 cups mixed vegetables (such as bell peppers, zucchini, and cherry tomatoes), chopped
- 2 tablespoons olive oil
- Salt and pepper to taste
- 1/4 cup fresh parsley, chopped
- 1/4 cup feta cheese, crumbled (optional)

For the vinaigrette:

- 3 tablespoons olive oil
- 2 tablespoons lemon juice
- 1 tablespoon balsamic vinegar
- 1 teaspoon Dijon mustard
- 1 teaspoon honey or maple syrup
- Salt and pepper to taste

Instructions:

1. Preheat the oven to 400°F (200°C).
2. In a saucepan, combine the quinoa and water or vegetable broth. Bring to a boil, then reduce the heat to low, cover, and simmer for 15-20 minutes, or until the quinoa is tender and the liquid is absorbed. Remove from heat and let it sit, covered, for 5 minutes. Fluff with a fork and set aside.
3. Meanwhile, toss the mixed vegetables with olive oil, salt, and pepper on a baking sheet. Roast in the preheated oven for 20-25 minutes, or until the vegetables are tender and lightly browned.
4. In a small bowl, whisk together the ingredients for the vinaigrette until well combined.
5. In a large bowl, combine the cooked quinoa, roasted vegetables, chickpeas, fresh parsley, and crumbled feta cheese (if using).
6. Pour the vinaigrette over the salad and toss until everything is evenly coated.
7. Serve the quinoa salad warm or chilled.

Nutritional Information: (per serving)

- Calories: 320 kcal
- Carbohydrates: 40g
- Protein: 10g
- Fat: 14g
- Fiber: 8g

3. Ginger-Lime Shrimp Tacos with Mango Salsa

Introduction: These ginger-lime shrimp tacos are bursting with fresh flavors and vibrant colors. Topped with a zesty mango salsa, they're a delightful combination of sweet, tangy, and spicy, perfect for a light and refreshing meal.

Total Prep Time: 30 minutes

Ingredients:

- 1 lb shrimp, peeled and deveined
- 2 tablespoons olive oil
- 2 cloves garlic, minced
- 1 tablespoon freshly grated ginger
- Zest and juice of 1 lime
- Salt and pepper to taste
- 8 small corn or flour tortillas
- 1 ripe mango, diced
- 1/2 red onion, finely chopped
- 1 jalapeño, seeded and minced
- 1/4 cup fresh cilantro, chopped
- 1 tablespoon lime juice
- Salt to taste
- Optional toppings: shredded cabbage, avocado slices, sour cream

Instructions:

1. In a bowl, combine the shrimp with olive oil, minced garlic, grated ginger, lime zest, lime juice, salt, and pepper. Let it marinate for 10-15 minutes.
2. Heat a skillet or grill pan over medium-high heat. Add the marinated shrimp and cook for 2-3 minutes per side, or until they turn pink and opaque. Remove from heat and set aside.
3. In a separate bowl, combine diced mango, chopped red onion, minced jalapeño, chopped cilantro, lime juice, and a pinch of salt. Mix well to combine.
4. Warm the tortillas in a dry skillet or microwave.
5. Assemble the tacos by placing a few shrimp on each tortilla, then topping with mango salsa and any desired additional toppings.
6. Serve the ginger-lime shrimp tacos immediately, accompanied by lime wedges.

Dr. Lukas Loewe

Nutritional Information: (per serving, without optional toppings)
- Calories: 250 kcal
- Carbohydrates: 30g
- Protein: 20g
- Fat: 6g
- Fiber: 3g

4. Magnesium-Packed Lentil Soup with Spinach and Turmeric

Introduction: This comforting lentil soup is not only delicious but also packed with magnesium-rich ingredients like lentils, spinach, and turmeric. Warm and nourishing, it's the perfect meal for chilly days or when you need a boost of energy.

Total Prep Time: 45 minutes

Ingredients:
- 1 cup dried green or brown lentils, rinsed and drained
- 1 tablespoon olive oil
- 1 onion, diced
- 2 carrots, diced
- 2 celery stalks, diced
- 3 cloves garlic, minced
- 1 teaspoon ground turmeric
- 1 teaspoon ground cumin
- 1/2 teaspoon ground coriander
- 6 cups vegetable broth
- 2 cups water
- 2 cups fresh spinach leaves
- Salt and pepper to taste
- Fresh lemon juice (optional)
- Chopped fresh parsley for garnish (optional)

Instructions:
1. In a large pot, heat olive oil over medium heat. Add diced onion, carrots, and celery, and sauté until softened, about 5 minutes.
2. Add minced garlic, ground turmeric, ground cumin, and ground coriander to the pot. Cook for another 1-2 minutes, until fragrant.
3. Stir in the dried lentils, vegetable broth, and water. Bring the soup to a boil, then reduce heat to low and let it

simmer, partially covered, for 25-30 minutes, or until the lentils are tender.

4. Add fresh spinach leaves to the soup and cook for an additional 2-3 minutes, until wilted.
5. Season the soup with salt and pepper to taste. If desired, add a squeeze of fresh lemon juice for brightness.
6. Ladle the lentil soup into bowls and garnish with chopped fresh parsley, if using.
7. Serve hot and enjoy this magnesium-packed lentil soup as a comforting meal.

Nutritional Information: (per serving)
- Calories: 200 kcal
- Carbohydrates: 30g
- Protein: 12g
- Fat: 3g
- Fiber: 10g

5. Ginger and Garlic Tofu Stir-Fry with Brown Rice

Introduction: This tofu stir-fry is a flavorful and nutritious dish that's quick and easy to make. The combination of ginger, garlic, and savory tofu pairs perfectly with crisp vegetables, all served over wholesome brown rice for a satisfying meal.

Total Prep Time: 25 minutes

Ingredients:
- 1 block (14 oz) extra-firm tofu, pressed and cubed
- 2 tablespoons soy sauce
- 1 tablespoon sesame oil
- 2 teaspoons freshly grated ginger
- 3 cloves garlic, minced
- 2 tablespoons vegetable oil
- 2 cups mixed vegetables (such as bell peppers, broccoli, and snap peas), sliced
- Cooked brown rice for serving
- Optional garnishes: sliced green onions, sesame seeds

Instructions:
1. In a bowl, combine the cubed tofu with soy sauce, sesame oil, grated ginger, and minced garlic. Let it marinate for 10-15 minutes.
2. Heat vegetable oil in a large skillet or wok over medium-high heat.

Dr. Lukas Loewe

3. Add the marinated tofu to the skillet and cook for 5-7 minutes, stirring occasionally, until golden brown and crispy on all sides. Remove the tofu from the skillet and set aside.
4. In the same skillet, add the mixed vegetables and stir-fry for 3-5 minutes, or until tender-crisp.
5. Return the cooked tofu to the skillet and toss everything together until heated through.
6. Serve the ginger and garlic tofu stir-fry hot over cooked brown rice.
7. Garnish with sliced green onions and sesame seeds, if desired.

Nutritional Information: (per serving, without rice)
- Calories: 250 kcal
- Carbohydrates: 15g
- Protein: 15g
- Fat: 15g
- Fiber: 5g

6. Magnesium-Boosting Greek Salad with Feta and Kalamata Olives

Introduction: This classic Greek salad is a refreshing and nutrient-packed dish that's bursting with Mediterranean flavors. Loaded with magnesium-rich ingredients like leafy greens, olives, and feta cheese, it's perfect for a light lunch or side dish.

Total Prep Time: 15 minutes

Ingredients:
- 4 cups mixed salad greens (such as romaine, spinach, and arugula)
- 1 cucumber, diced
- 1 cup cherry tomatoes, halved
- 1/2 red onion, thinly sliced
- 1/2 cup Kalamata olives, pitted
- 1/2 cup crumbled feta cheese
- 2 tablespoons extra-virgin olive oil
- 1 tablespoon red wine vinegar
- 1 teaspoon dried oregano
- Salt and pepper to taste

Instructions:

1. In a large salad bowl, combine the mixed salad greens, diced cucumber, halved cherry tomatoes, thinly sliced red onion, pitted Kalamata olives, and crumbled feta cheese.
2. In a small bowl, whisk together the extra-virgin olive oil, red wine vinegar, dried oregano, salt, and pepper to make the dressing.
3. Drizzle the dressing over the salad and toss gently to coat all the ingredients evenly.
4. Serve the magnesium-boosting Greek salad immediately as a light and refreshing meal or side dish.

Nutritional Information: (per serving)
- Calories: 200 kcal
- Carbohydrates: 10g
- Protein: 5g
- Fat: 15g
- Fiber: 3g

7. Ginger-Soy Glazed Salmon Salad with Avocado and Edamame

Introduction: This ginger-soy glazed salmon salad is a delicious and nutritious meal that's perfect for lunch or a light dinner. Tender, flavorful salmon is paired with creamy avocado and protein-rich edamame, all tossed with a zesty ginger-soy dressing for a burst of Asian-inspired flavors.

Total Prep Time: 25 minutes

Ingredients:
- 2 salmon fillets (6 oz each), skin-on
- 2 tablespoons soy sauce
- 1 tablespoon honey or maple syrup
- 1 teaspoon freshly grated ginger
- 2 cups mixed salad greens
- 1 avocado, sliced
- 1/2 cup shelled edamame, cooked
- 1 tablespoon sesame seeds, toasted
- Optional garnishes: sliced green onions, cilantro leaves

For the ginger-soy dressing:
- 2 tablespoons soy sauce
- 1 tablespoon rice vinegar
- 1 tablespoon sesame oil
- 1 teaspoon freshly grated ginger

- 1 teaspoon honey or maple syrup
- 1 garlic clove, minced

Instructions:

1. Preheat the oven to 400°F (200°C). Line a baking sheet with parchment paper.
2. In a small bowl, whisk together soy sauce, honey or maple syrup, and freshly grated ginger to make the glaze.
3. Place the salmon fillets skin-side down on the prepared baking sheet. Brush the glaze over the salmon.
4. Bake in the preheated oven for 12-15 minutes, or until the salmon is cooked through and flakes easily with a fork.
5. While the salmon is baking, prepare the ginger-soy dressing by whisking together soy sauce, rice vinegar, sesame oil, freshly grated ginger, honey or maple syrup, and minced garlic in a small bowl.
6. In a large salad bowl, combine mixed salad greens, sliced avocado, cooked edamame, and toasted sesame seeds.
7. Once the salmon is cooked, flake it into large chunks and add it to the salad bowl.
8. Drizzle the ginger-soy dressing over the salad and toss gently to coat.
9. Garnish the salad with sliced green onions and cilantro leaves, if desired.
10. Serve the ginger-soy glazed salmon salad immediately as a satisfying and flavorful meal.

Nutritional Information: (per serving)

- Calories: 400 kcal
- Carbohydrates: 15g
- Protein: 30g
- Fat: 25g
- Fiber: 7g

8. Magnesium-Rich Black Bean and Sweet Potato Quesadillas

Introduction: These black bean and sweet potato quesadillas are a delicious and satisfying vegetarian meal that's packed with magnesium-rich ingredients. Creamy black beans, sweet roasted sweet potatoes, and gooey melted cheese are sandwiched between crispy tortillas for a flavor-packed bite.

Total Prep Time: 35 minutes

Ingredients:

- 1 large sweet potato, peeled and diced
- 1 tablespoon olive oil
- 1 teaspoon ground cumin
- 1/2 teaspoon smoked paprika
- Salt and pepper to taste
- 4 large flour tortillas
- 1 can (15 oz) black beans, drained and rinsed
- 1 cup shredded cheese (cheddar, Monterey Jack, or Mexican blend)
- Optional toppings: salsa, sour cream, avocado slices, cilantro

Instructions:

1. Preheat the oven to 400°F (200°C). Line a baking sheet with parchment paper.
2. In a bowl, toss the diced sweet potato with olive oil, ground cumin, smoked paprika, salt, and pepper until evenly coated.
3. Spread the seasoned sweet potato cubes in a single layer on the prepared baking sheet.
4. Roast in the preheated oven for 20-25 minutes, or until the sweet potatoes are tender and lightly browned.
5. In a large skillet, warm one flour tortilla over medium heat for about 1 minute on each side, until lightly toasted.
6. Spread a layer of black beans on half of the toasted tortilla, then top with roasted sweet potato cubes and shredded cheese.
7. Fold the tortilla in half to cover the filling, creating a half-moon shape.
8. Cook the quesadilla in the skillet for 2-3 minutes on each side, until the cheese is melted and the tortilla is golden brown and crispy.
9. Remove the quesadilla from the skillet and repeat with the remaining tortillas and filling ingredients.
10. Cut the quesadillas into wedges and serve hot with optional toppings like salsa, sour cream, avocado slices, and cilantro.

Nutritional Information: (per serving, without toppings)
- Calories: 350 kcal

Dr. Lukas Loewe

- Carbohydrates: 45g
- Protein: 15g
- Fat: 12g
- Fiber: 8g

9. Ginger-Chicken Lettuce Wraps with Cashews and Water Chestnuts

Introduction: These ginger-chicken lettuce wraps are a light and flavorful meal that's perfect for a quick lunch or dinner. Tender chicken cooked with aromatic ginger, crunchy water chestnuts, and creamy cashews are served in crisp lettuce cups for a refreshing and satisfying dish.

Total Prep Time: 25 minutes

Ingredients:
- 1 lb ground chicken
- 2 tablespoons vegetable oil
- 2 cloves garlic, minced
- 1 tablespoon freshly grated ginger
- 1/4 cup soy sauce
- 2 tablespoons hoisin sauce
- 1 tablespoon rice vinegar
- 1 teaspoon sesame oil
- 1 can (8 oz) water chestnuts, drained and diced
- 1/4 cup cashews, chopped
- 1/4 cup green onions, thinly sliced
- 1 head iceberg or butter lettuce, leaves separated
- Optional garnishes: chopped cilantro, sliced red chili

Instructions:
1. Heat vegetable oil in a large skillet or wok over medium-high heat.
2. Add minced garlic and grated ginger to the skillet and cook for 1 minute, until fragrant.
3. Add ground chicken to the skillet and cook, breaking it apart with a spoon, until browned and cooked through.
4. In a small bowl, whisk together soy sauce, hoisin sauce, rice vinegar, and sesame oil. Pour the sauce over the cooked chicken in the skillet.

5. Stir in diced water chestnuts, chopped cashews, and sliced green onions. Cook for another 2-3 minutes, until heated through.
6. To serve, spoon the ginger-chicken mixture into individual lettuce leaves, creating lettuce wraps.
7. Garnish the lettuce wraps with chopped cilantro and sliced red chili, if desired.
8. Serve the ginger-chicken lettuce wraps immediately, with extra sauce on the side for dipping.

Nutritional Information: (per serving, based on 4 servings)
- Calories: 300 kcal
- Carbohydrates: 12g
- Protein: 20g
- Fat: 20g
- Fiber: 3g

10. Magnesium-Infused Kale and Quinoa Salad with Lemon-Tahini Dressing

Introduction: This kale and quinoa salad is a nutrient-packed dish that's both delicious and satisfying. Packed with magnesium-rich ingredients like kale, quinoa, and almonds, and drizzled with a creamy lemon-tahini dressing, it's a perfect meal for boosting energy and supporting overall health.

Total Prep Time: 30 minutes

Ingredients:
- 1 cup quinoa, rinsed
- 2 cups water or vegetable broth
- 4 cups kale, stemmed and finely chopped
- 1/4 cup almonds, chopped
- 1/4 cup dried cranberries or raisins
- 1/4 cup crumbled feta cheese (optional)
- Salt and pepper to taste

For the lemon-tahini dressing:
- 3 tablespoons tahini
- 2 tablespoons lemon juice
- 1 tablespoon olive oil
- 1 tablespoon water
- 1 teaspoon honey or maple syrup
- 1 clove garlic, minced
- Salt and pepper to taste

Instructions:

1. In a saucepan, combine the quinoa and water or vegetable broth. Bring to a boil, then reduce the heat to low, cover, and simmer for 15-20 minutes, or until the quinoa is tender and the liquid is absorbed. Remove from heat and let it sit, covered, for 5 minutes. Fluff with a fork and set aside to cool.
2. In a large mixing bowl, combine the chopped kale, cooked quinoa, chopped almonds, and dried cranberries or raisins.
3. In a small bowl, whisk together the ingredients for the lemon-tahini dressing until smooth and well combined.
4. Pour the dressing over the kale and quinoa mixture, and toss until everything is evenly coated.
5. Season with salt and pepper to taste. If using, sprinkle crumbled feta cheese over the salad.
6. Serve the magnesium-infused kale and quinoa salad immediately, or refrigerate for later. This salad can be enjoyed cold or at room temperature.

Nutritional Information: (per serving, based on 4 servings)

- Calories: 300 kcal
- Carbohydrates: 30g
- Protein: 9g
- Fat: 17g
- Fiber: 5g

11. Spicy Ginger Beef Noodle Bowl with Bok Choy

Introduction: This spicy ginger beef noodle bowl is a satisfying and flavorful dish that's perfect for a cozy dinner. Tender strips of beef are cooked with aromatic ginger and spicy chili sauce, then served over noodles and crisp bok choy for a delicious and comforting meal.

Total Prep Time: 35 minutes

Ingredients:

- 8 oz flank steak, thinly sliced
- 2 tablespoons soy sauce
- 1 tablespoon sesame oil
- 2 teaspoons cornstarch
- 2 tablespoons vegetable oil
- 2 cloves garlic, minced

- 1 tablespoon freshly grated ginger
- 1 teaspoon chili flakes (adjust to taste)
- 4 cups cooked noodles (such as udon or rice noodles)
- 2 baby bok choy, halved
- 2 green onions, thinly sliced
- Sesame seeds for garnish
- Lime wedges for serving

Instructions:

1. In a bowl, combine the sliced flank steak with soy sauce, sesame oil, and cornstarch. Toss to coat the beef evenly and set aside to marinate for 10-15 minutes.
2. Heat vegetable oil in a large skillet or wok over high heat.
3. Add minced garlic, grated ginger, and chili flakes to the skillet and stir-fry for 1-2 minutes, until fragrant.
4. Add the marinated beef to the skillet and cook, stirring constantly, until browned and cooked to your desired level of doneness.
5. Meanwhile, blanch the halved baby bok choy in boiling water for 2-3 minutes, or until tender-crisp. Drain and set aside.
6. To assemble the noodle bowls, divide the cooked noodles among serving bowls. Top with the cooked beef and bok choy.
7. Garnish with sliced green onions and sesame seeds.
8. Serve the spicy ginger beef noodle bowls hot, with lime wedges on the side for squeezing over the dish.

Nutritional Information: (per serving)

- Calories: 400 kcal
- Carbohydrates: 35g
- Protein: 25g
- Fat: 18g
- Fiber: 5g

12. Magnesium-Packed Chickpea and Spinach Curry with Basmati Rice

Introduction: This chickpea and spinach curry is a comforting and flavorful dish that's loaded with magnesium-rich ingredients. Tender chickpeas and wilted spinach are simmered in a fragrant curry sauce, then served over fluffy basmati rice for a delicious and nutritious meal.

Total Prep Time: 40 minutes
Ingredients:
- 1 tablespoon vegetable oil
- 1 onion, finely chopped
- 2 cloves garlic, minced
- 1 tablespoon freshly grated ginger
- 1 tablespoon curry powder
- 1 teaspoon ground turmeric
- 1/2 teaspoon ground cumin
- 1/2 teaspoon ground coriander
- 1 can (15 oz) chickpeas, drained and rinsed
- 1 can (14 oz) diced tomatoes
- 1 can (14 oz) coconut milk
- 4 cups fresh spinach leaves
- Salt and pepper to taste
- Cooked basmati rice for serving

Instructions:
1. Heat vegetable oil in a large skillet or pot over medium heat.
2. Add chopped onion, minced garlic, and grated ginger to the skillet. Cook, stirring occasionally, for 3-4 minutes, until softened and fragrant.
3. Stir in curry powder, ground turmeric, ground cumin, and ground coriander. Cook for another minute, until spices are toasted and fragrant.
4. Add drained chickpeas, diced tomatoes (with their juices), and coconut milk to the skillet. Stir to combine.
5. Bring the curry to a simmer, then reduce the heat to low and let it cook for 15-20 minutes, stirring occasionally, until the sauce thickens slightly.
6. Stir in fresh spinach leaves and cook for an additional 2-3 minutes, until wilted.
7. Season the curry with salt and pepper to taste.
8. Serve the magnesium-packed chickpea and spinach curry hot, over cooked basmati rice.

Nutritional Information: (per serving, curry only)
- Calories: 300 kcal
- Carbohydrates: 20g
- Protein: 10g
- Fat: 20g

- Fiber: 5g

13. Ginger-Sesame Soba Noodle Salad with Cucumber and Carrots

Introduction: This ginger-sesame soba noodle salad is a refreshing and flavorful dish that's perfect for a light lunch or dinner. Chewy soba noodles are tossed with crunchy cucumber, carrots, and a zesty ginger-sesame dressing for a satisfying and nutritious meal.

Total Prep Time: 20 minutes

Ingredients:
- 8 oz soba noodles
- 1 cucumber, julienned
- 2 carrots, julienned
- 1/4 cup fresh cilantro leaves, chopped
- 2 tablespoons sesame seeds, toasted
- Optional garnishes: sliced green onions, chopped peanuts

For the ginger-sesame dressing:
- 2 tablespoons soy sauce
- 1 tablespoon rice vinegar
- 1 tablespoon sesame oil
- 1 tablespoon honey or maple syrup
- 1 tablespoon freshly grated ginger
- 1 clove garlic, minced
- 1 teaspoon sriracha or chili garlic sauce (optional)

Instructions:
1. Cook the soba noodles according to the package instructions. Drain and rinse under cold water to stop the cooking process. Set aside.
2. In a large mixing bowl, combine the cooked soba noodles, julienned cucumber, julienned carrots, chopped cilantro leaves, and toasted sesame seeds.
3. In a small bowl, whisk together the ingredients for the ginger-sesame dressing until well combined.
4. Pour the dressing over the soba noodle mixture and toss until everything is evenly coated.
5. Garnish the ginger-sesame soba noodle salad with sliced green onions and chopped peanuts, if desired.
6. Serve the salad immediately as a refreshing and nutritious meal, or refrigerate for later.

Nutritional Information: (per serving, based on 4 servings)
- Calories: 250 kcal
- Carbohydrates: 40g
- Protein: 8g
- Fat: 6g
- Fiber: 4g

14. Magnesium-Rich Tuna Salad Stuffed Avocados

Introduction: These tuna salad stuffed avocados are a simple yet satisfying meal that's packed with magnesium-rich ingredients. Creamy avocado halves are filled with a flavorful tuna salad made with crunchy celery, tangy lemon juice, and creamy Greek yogurt for a delicious and nutritious dish.

Total Prep Time: 15 minutes

Ingredients:
- 2 ripe avocados, halved and pitted
- 1 can (5 oz) tuna, drained
- 2 tablespoons Greek yogurt
- 1 tablespoon lemon juice
- 1 celery stalk, finely chopped
- 1 tablespoon red onion, finely chopped
- Salt and pepper to taste
- Optional garnishes: chopped parsley, paprika

Instructions:
1. In a mixing bowl, combine drained tuna, Greek yogurt, lemon juice, chopped celery, and chopped red onion. Mix well to combine.
2. Season the tuna salad with salt and pepper to taste.
3. Scoop out a portion of the avocado flesh from each avocado half to create a larger cavity for the filling.
4. Divide the tuna salad evenly among the avocado halves, mounding it on top.
5. Garnish the stuffed avocados with chopped parsley and a sprinkle of paprika, if desired.
6. Serve the magnesium-rich tuna salad stuffed avocados immediately as a light and satisfying meal.

Nutritional Information: (per serving, based on 1 stuffed avocado half)
- Calories: 200 kcal

- Carbohydrates: 10g
- Protein: 10g
- Fat: 15g
- Fiber: 7g

15. Ginger and Turmeric Veggie Wrap with Hummus

Introduction: This ginger and turmeric veggie wrap with hummus is a flavorful and nutritious meal that's perfect for a quick lunch or on-the-go snack. Vibrant vegetables, aromatic spices, and creamy hummus are wrapped in a soft tortilla for a delicious and satisfying bite.

Total Prep Time: 15 minutes

Ingredients:
- 4 large flour tortillas
- 1/2 cup hummus
- 1 bell pepper, thinly sliced
- 1 cucumber, julienned
- 1 carrot, julienned
- 1/4 red cabbage, thinly sliced
- 1 tablespoon freshly grated ginger
- 1 teaspoon ground turmeric
- Salt and pepper to taste
- Optional add-ins: avocado slices, sprouts, shredded lettuce

Instructions:
1. Lay out the flour tortillas on a clean work surface.
2. Spread a generous layer of hummus evenly over each tortilla.
3. Arrange sliced bell pepper, julienned cucumber, julienned carrot, and thinly sliced red cabbage on top of the hummus layer.
4. Sprinkle freshly grated ginger and ground turmeric over the vegetables.
5. Season with salt and pepper to taste.
6. Add optional add-ins like avocado slices, sprouts, or shredded lettuce if desired.
7. Roll up each tortilla tightly to enclose the filling, creating a wrap.
8. Slice the wraps in half diagonally, if desired, and serve immediately.

Nutritional Information: (per serving, based on 1 wrap)

- Calories: 250 kcal
- Carbohydrates: 30g
- Protein: 6g
- Fat: 12g
- Fiber: 5g

16. Magnesium-Boosting Spinach and Lentil Salad with Roasted Beets

Introduction: This spinach and lentil salad with roasted beets is a nutritious and satisfying dish that's bursting with flavor and packed with magnesium-rich ingredients. Tender lentils, earthy roasted beets, and fresh spinach are tossed in a tangy balsamic vinaigrette for a delicious and colorful salad.

Total Prep Time: 40 minutes

Ingredients:
- 1 cup green or brown lentils
- 2 medium beets, peeled and diced
- 2 tablespoons olive oil, divided
- Salt and pepper to taste
- 4 cups fresh spinach leaves
- 1/4 cup crumbled goat cheese or feta cheese
- 1/4 cup chopped walnuts, toasted
- Optional garnish: fresh parsley

For the balsamic vinaigrette:
- 3 tablespoons balsamic vinegar
- 2 tablespoons olive oil
- 1 teaspoon Dijon mustard
- 1 teaspoon honey or maple syrup
- Salt and pepper to taste

Instructions:
1. Preheat the oven to 400°F (200°C). Line a baking sheet with parchment paper.
2. In a bowl, toss diced beets with 1 tablespoon olive oil, salt, and pepper until evenly coated.
3. Spread the seasoned beets in a single layer on the prepared baking sheet.
4. Roast in the preheated oven for 20-25 minutes, or until the beets are tender and caramelized.

5. Meanwhile, rinse the lentils under cold water and drain. Cook the lentils according to the package instructions until tender, then drain any excess water and set aside to cool.
6. In a small bowl, whisk together balsamic vinegar, olive oil, Dijon mustard, honey or maple syrup, salt, and pepper to make the vinaigrette.
7. In a large mixing bowl, combine cooked lentils, roasted beets, fresh spinach leaves, crumbled goat cheese or feta cheese, and chopped toasted walnuts.
8. Drizzle the balsamic vinaigrette over the salad and toss gently to coat.
9. Garnish the salad with fresh parsley, if desired.
10. Serve the magnesium-boosting spinach and lentil salad immediately as a nutritious and flavorful meal.

Nutritional Information: (per serving, based on 4 servings)
- Calories: 300 kcal
- Carbohydrates: 30g
- Protein: 10g
- Fat: 15g
- Fiber: 8g

17. Gingered Butternut Squash and Coconut Soup

Introduction: This gingered butternut squash and coconut soup is a comforting and flavorful dish that's perfect for cooler weather. Creamy butternut squash is infused with aromatic ginger and coconut milk, then pureed until smooth for a velvety soup that's sure to warm you up from the inside out.

Total Prep Time: 45 minutes

Ingredients:
- 1 medium butternut squash, peeled, seeded, and diced
- 1 tablespoon olive oil
- 1 onion, chopped
- 2 cloves garlic, minced
- 1 tablespoon freshly grated ginger
- 4 cups vegetable broth
- 1 can (14 oz) coconut milk
- Salt and pepper to taste
- Optional garnishes: toasted pumpkin seeds, chopped fresh cilantro, drizzle of coconut milk

Instructions:

1. In a large pot or Dutch oven, heat olive oil over medium heat.
2. Add chopped onion and minced garlic to the pot. Cook, stirring occasionally, for 3-4 minutes, until softened.
3. Stir in freshly grated ginger and cook for another minute, until fragrant.
4. Add diced butternut squash to the pot, along with vegetable broth. Bring to a boil, then reduce the heat to low and let the soup simmer for 20-25 minutes, or until the squash is tender.
5. Once the squash is cooked through, remove the pot from heat and let it cool slightly.
6. Using an immersion blender or regular blender, puree the soup until smooth and creamy.
7. Return the pot to the stove over low heat. Stir in coconut milk until well combined.
8. Season the soup with salt and pepper to taste.
9. Serve the gingered butternut squash and coconut soup hot, garnished with toasted pumpkin seeds, chopped fresh cilantro, and a drizzle of coconut milk, if desired.

Nutritional Information: (per serving, based on 6 servings)
- Calories: 200 kcal
- Carbohydrates: 20g
- Protein: 3g
- Fat: 14g
- Fiber: 3g

18. Magnesium-Packed Mediterranean Couscous Salad with Olives and Feta

Introduction: This Mediterranean couscous salad is a vibrant and flavorful dish that's perfect for a light lunch or side dish. Nutty couscous is tossed with colorful vegetables, briny olives, tangy feta cheese, and a zesty lemon-herb dressing for a delicious and satisfying salad.

Total Prep Time: 30 minutes

Ingredients:
- 1 cup couscous
- 1 1/4 cups vegetable broth or water
- 1 tablespoon olive oil
- 1 cucumber, diced

- 1 bell pepper, diced
- 1/2 red onion, finely chopped
- 1/2 cup cherry tomatoes, halved
- 1/4 cup Kalamata olives, pitted and chopped
- 1/4 cup crumbled feta cheese
- 2 tablespoons chopped fresh parsley
- Salt and pepper to taste

For the lemon-herb dressing:
- 3 tablespoons olive oil
- 2 tablespoons lemon juice
- 1 teaspoon honey or maple syrup
- 1 clove garlic, minced
- 1 teaspoon dried oregano
- Salt and pepper to taste

Instructions:
1. In a saucepan, bring vegetable broth or water to a boil. Stir in couscous and olive oil. Cover, remove from heat, and let it sit for 5 minutes, or until the liquid is absorbed. Fluff with a fork and set aside to cool.
2. In a large mixing bowl, combine cooked couscous, diced cucumber, diced bell pepper, finely chopped red onion, halved cherry tomatoes, chopped Kalamata olives, crumbled feta cheese, and chopped fresh parsley.
3. In a small bowl, whisk together olive oil, lemon juice, honey or maple syrup, minced garlic, dried oregano, salt, and pepper to make the lemon-herb dressing.
4. Pour the dressing over the couscous salad and toss gently to coat everything evenly.
5. Season with additional salt and pepper to taste, if needed.
6. Serve the magnesium-packed Mediterranean couscous salad immediately as a delicious and colorful dish.

Nutritional Information: (per serving, based on 6 servings)
- Calories: 250 kcal
- Carbohydrates: 30g
- Protein: 6g
- Fat: 12g
- Fiber: 3g

19. Ginger and Garlic Beef Lettuce Cups with Jasmine Rice

Introduction: These ginger and garlic beef lettuce cups with jasmine rice are a flavorful and satisfying meal that's perfect for a light dinner or appetizer. Tender beef stir-fried with aromatic ginger and garlic is served in crisp lettuce cups and accompanied by fragrant jasmine rice for a delicious and balanced dish.

Total Prep Time: 30 minutes

Ingredients:

- 1 cup jasmine rice
- 2 cups water
- 1 tablespoon vegetable oil
- 1 lb ground beef
- 2 cloves garlic, minced
- 1 tablespoon freshly grated ginger
- 2 tablespoons soy sauce
- 1 tablespoon hoisin sauce
- 1 teaspoon sesame oil
- 1 teaspoon rice vinegar
- 1/4 cup chopped green onions
- Salt and pepper to taste
- Butter lettuce leaves for serving

Instructions:

1. Rinse jasmine rice under cold water until the water runs clear. In a saucepan, combine the rinsed rice and water. Bring to a boil, then reduce the heat to low, cover, and simmer for 15-20 minutes, or until the rice is tender and the water is absorbed. Remove from heat and let it sit, covered, for 5 minutes. Fluff with a fork and set aside.
2. Heat vegetable oil in a large skillet or wok over medium-high heat.
3. Add ground beef to the skillet and cook, breaking it apart with a spoon, until browned and cooked through.
4. Add minced garlic and grated ginger to the skillet. Cook for 1-2 minutes, until fragrant.
5. In a small bowl, whisk together soy sauce, hoisin sauce, sesame oil, and rice vinegar. Pour the sauce over the cooked beef in the skillet.
6. Stir in chopped green onions and cook for another 2-3 minutes, until heated through.

7. Season with salt and pepper to taste.
8. To serve, spoon the ginger and garlic beef mixture into individual butter lettuce leaves, creating lettuce cups.
9. Serve the lettuce cups with jasmine rice on the side for a delicious and balanced meal.

Nutritional Information: (per serving, based on 4 servings)
- Calories: 350 kcal
- Carbohydrates: 40g
- Protein: 20g
- Fat: 12g
- Fiber: 2g

20. Magnesium-Rich Roasted Vegetable and Quinoa Buddha Bowl

Introduction: This magnesium-rich roasted vegetable and quinoa Buddha bowl is a wholesome and nourishing meal that's packed with flavor and nutrients. Oven-roasted vegetables, protein-rich quinoa, creamy avocado, and tangy tahini dressing come together to create a satisfying and balanced dish that's perfect for lunch or dinner.

Total Prep Time: 40 minutes

Ingredients:
- 1 cup quinoa, rinsed
- 2 cups water or vegetable broth
- 1 small sweet potato, peeled and diced
- 1 small zucchini, diced
- 1 red bell pepper, diced
- 1 cup cherry tomatoes
- 2 tablespoons olive oil
- Salt and pepper to taste
- 1 avocado, sliced
- 1/4 cup chopped fresh cilantro or parsley
- Optional garnish: toasted pumpkin seeds

For the tahini dressing:
- 1/4 cup tahini
- 2 tablespoons lemon juice
- 1 tablespoon olive oil
- 1 clove garlic, minced
- 1 teaspoon honey or maple syrup
- Salt and pepper to taste

Instructions:

1. Preheat the oven to 400°F (200°C). Line a baking sheet with parchment paper.
2. In a saucepan, combine quinoa and water or vegetable broth. Bring to a boil, then reduce the heat to low, cover, and simmer for 15-20 minutes, or until the quinoa is tender and the liquid is absorbed. Remove from heat and let it sit, covered, for 5 minutes. Fluff with a fork and set aside.
3. Meanwhile, spread diced sweet potato, diced zucchini, diced red bell pepper, and cherry tomatoes on the prepared baking sheet.
4. Drizzle olive oil over the vegetables and toss to coat evenly. Season with salt and pepper to taste.
5. Roast in the preheated oven for 20-25 minutes, or until the vegetables are tender and lightly caramelized.
6. In a small bowl, whisk together tahini, lemon juice, olive oil, minced garlic, honey or maple syrup, salt, and pepper to make the tahini dressing.
7. To assemble the Buddha bowls, divide cooked quinoa among serving bowls. Top with roasted vegetables, sliced avocado, and chopped fresh cilantro or parsley.
8. Drizzle tahini dressing over the Buddha bowls and sprinkle with toasted pumpkin seeds, if desired.
9. Serve the magnesium-rich roasted vegetable and quinoa Buddha bowls immediately as a wholesome and nourishing meal.

Nutritional Information: (per serving, based on 4 servings)

- Calories: 400 kcal
- Carbohydrates: 40g
- Protein: 10g
- Fat: 25g
- Fiber: 8g

6.3 Dinner Recipes:

1. Ginger and Garlic Shrimp Stir-Fry with Snow Peas and Bell Peppers

Introduction: This ginger and garlic shrimp stir-fry is a quick and flavorful dish that's perfect for busy weeknights. Succulent shrimp are cooked with aromatic ginger, garlic, crisp snow peas, and colorful bell peppers for a delicious and nutritious meal that's ready in minutes.

Total Prep Time: 20 minutes

Ingredients:
- 1 lb shrimp, peeled and deveined
- 2 tablespoons vegetable oil
- 3 cloves garlic, minced
- 1 tablespoon freshly grated ginger
- 1 cup snow peas, trimmed
- 1 bell pepper, thinly sliced
- 2 tablespoons soy sauce
- 1 tablespoon oyster sauce
- 1 teaspoon sesame oil
- Optional garnish: chopped green onions, sesame seeds

Instructions:
1. Heat vegetable oil in a large skillet or wok over high heat.
2. Add minced garlic and grated ginger to the skillet and cook for 1 minute, until fragrant.
3. Add shrimp to the skillet and cook for 2-3 minutes, until pink and cooked through. Remove the shrimp from the skillet and set aside.
4. In the same skillet, add snow peas and sliced bell pepper. Stir-fry for 2-3 minutes, until crisp-tender.
5. Return the cooked shrimp to the skillet.
6. In a small bowl, whisk together soy sauce, oyster sauce, and sesame oil. Pour the sauce over the shrimp and vegetables in the skillet.
7. Stir-fry everything together for another minute, until heated through and evenly coated with the sauce.
8. Garnish the ginger and garlic shrimp stir-fry with chopped green onions and sesame seeds, if desired.
9. Serve the stir-fry immediately over steamed rice or noodles.

Nutritional Information: (per serving, based on 4 servings)
- Calories: 200 kcal
- Carbohydrates: 6g
- Protein: 25g
- Fat: 8g

- Fiber: 2g

2. Magnesium-Rich Baked Salmon with Lemon and Dill

Introduction: This baked salmon with lemon and dill is a simple yet elegant dish that's bursting with flavor and packed with magnesium-rich ingredients. Tender salmon fillets are seasoned with zesty lemon, fragrant dill, and a hint of garlic, then baked to perfection for a delicious and nutritious meal.

Total Prep Time: 25 minutes

Ingredients:
- 4 salmon fillets (6 oz each)
- 2 tablespoons olive oil
- 2 cloves garlic, minced
- 2 tablespoons fresh lemon juice
- 1 tablespoon chopped fresh dill
- Salt and pepper to taste
- Lemon slices for garnish
- Fresh dill sprigs for garnish

Instructions:
1. Preheat the oven to 375°F (190°C). Line a baking sheet with parchment paper.
2. Place the salmon fillets on the prepared baking sheet.
3. In a small bowl, whisk together olive oil, minced garlic, lemon juice, and chopped fresh dill.
4. Drizzle the lemon-dill mixture over the salmon fillets, spreading it evenly to coat.
5. Season the salmon fillets with salt and pepper to taste.
6. Place lemon slices on top of each salmon fillet for extra flavor.
7. Bake the salmon in the preheated oven for 12-15 minutes, or until the fish is cooked through and flakes easily with a fork.
8. Once cooked, remove the salmon from the oven and garnish with fresh dill sprigs.
9. Serve the magnesium-rich baked salmon with lemon and dill hot, with your favorite side dishes.

Nutritional Information: (per serving, based on 4 servings)
- Calories: 300 kcal
- Carbohydrates: 1g
- Protein: 25g

Dr. Lukas Loewe

- Fat: 22g
- Fiber: 0g

3. Ginger-Coconut Chicken Curry with Jasmine Rice

Introduction: This ginger-coconut chicken curry is a comforting and aromatic dish that's packed with flavor and nutrients. Tender chicken pieces are simmered in a rich and creamy coconut curry sauce infused with ginger, garlic, and warm spices, then served over fragrant jasmine rice for a satisfying meal that will warm you from the inside out.

Total Prep Time: 45 minutes

Ingredients:
- 1 lb boneless, skinless chicken breasts, cut into bite-sized pieces
- 2 tablespoons vegetable oil
- 1 onion, finely chopped
- 3 cloves garlic, minced
- 1 tablespoon freshly grated ginger
- 2 tablespoons curry powder
- 1 teaspoon ground turmeric
- 1 teaspoon ground coriander
- 1/2 teaspoon ground cumin
- 1 can (14 oz) coconut milk
- 1 cup chicken broth
- 2 cups diced tomatoes (fresh or canned)
- Salt and pepper to taste
- Fresh cilantro for garnish
- Cooked jasmine rice for serving

Instructions:
1. In a large skillet or pot, heat vegetable oil over medium heat.
2. Add finely chopped onion to the skillet and cook for 5-6 minutes, until softened and translucent.
3. Stir in minced garlic and freshly grated ginger, and cook for another minute, until fragrant.
4. Add curry powder, ground turmeric, ground coriander, and ground cumin to the skillet. Stir to combine with the onion mixture and cook for 1-2 minutes, until spices are toasted.

5. Add bite-sized chicken pieces to the skillet and cook until browned on all sides.
6. Pour in coconut milk, chicken broth, and diced tomatoes. Stir to combine and bring the mixture to a simmer.
7. Reduce the heat to low and let the curry simmer, uncovered, for 20-25 minutes, stirring occasionally, until the chicken is cooked through and the sauce has thickened slightly.
8. Season the ginger-coconut chicken curry with salt and pepper to taste.
9. Serve the curry hot over cooked jasmine rice, garnished with fresh cilantro.

Nutritional Information: (per serving, curry only)
- Calories: 350 kcal
- Carbohydrates: 12g
- Protein: 25g
- Fat: 24g
- Fiber: 3g

4. Magnesium-Infused Vegetable Stir-Fry with Tofu

Introduction: This magnesium-infused vegetable stir-fry with tofu is a colorful and nutritious dish that's quick and easy to make. Crisp and vibrant vegetables are stir-fried with protein-rich tofu and tossed in a flavorful sauce infused with ginger and garlic for a delicious and satisfying meal.

Total Prep Time: 30 minutes

Ingredients:
- 1 block (14 oz) firm tofu, drained and pressed
- 2 tablespoons soy sauce
- 1 tablespoon cornstarch
- 2 tablespoons vegetable oil
- 2 cloves garlic, minced
- 1 tablespoon freshly grated ginger
- 1 bell pepper, thinly sliced
- 1 cup broccoli florets
- 1 carrot, thinly sliced
- 1 cup snow peas, trimmed
- 1/4 cup low-sodium vegetable broth
- 2 tablespoons oyster sauce

- 1 tablespoon hoisin sauce
- Cooked rice or noodles for serving

Instructions:
1. Cut pressed tofu into cubes and place them in a bowl. Toss with soy sauce and cornstarch until evenly coated.
2. Heat vegetable oil in a large skillet or wok over medium-high heat.
3. Add minced garlic and freshly grated ginger to the skillet and cook for 1 minute, until fragrant.
4. Add tofu cubes to the skillet in a single layer and cook for 3-4 minutes on each side, until golden and crispy. Remove tofu from the skillet and set aside.
5. In the same skillet, add bell pepper, broccoli florets, carrot slices, and snow peas. Stir-fry for 4-5 minutes, until vegetables are tender-crisp.
6. In a small bowl, whisk together low-sodium vegetable broth, oyster sauce, and hoisin sauce. Pour the sauce mixture over the vegetables in the skillet.
7. Return the cooked tofu to the skillet and toss everything together until evenly coated with the sauce.
8. Cook for another 1-2 minutes, until heated through.
9. Serve the magnesium-infused vegetable stir-fry with tofu hot, over cooked rice or noodles.

Nutritional Information: (per serving, stir-fry only)
- Calories: 250 kcal
- Carbohydrates: 15g
- Protein: 15g
- Fat: 15g
- Fiber: 5g

5. Ginger-Soy Glazed Cod with Sesame Broccoli

Introduction: This ginger-soy glazed cod with sesame broccoli is a healthy and flavorful dish that's perfect for a weeknight dinner. Tender cod fillets are marinated in a zesty ginger-soy sauce, then baked to perfection and served with crisp sesame broccoli for a delicious and nutritious meal.

Total Prep Time: 30 minutes

Ingredients:
- 4 cod fillets (6 oz each)
- 1/4 cup soy sauce

- 2 tablespoons honey or maple syrup
- 1 tablespoon freshly grated ginger
- 2 cloves garlic, minced
- 1 tablespoon sesame oil
- 2 tablespoons sesame seeds
- 1 lb broccoli florets
- 2 tablespoons olive oil
- Salt and pepper to taste
- Cooked rice or quinoa for serving

Instructions:
1. Preheat the oven to 400°F (200°C). Line a baking sheet with parchment paper.
2. In a small bowl, whisk together soy sauce, honey or maple syrup, freshly grated ginger, minced garlic, and sesame oil to make the ginger-soy glaze.
3. Place cod fillets on the prepared baking sheet. Brush each fillet generously with the ginger-soy glaze.
4. Sprinkle sesame seeds over the glazed cod fillets.
5. Bake the cod in the preheated oven for 12-15 minutes, or until fish is cooked through and flakes easily with a fork.
6. While the cod is baking, prepare the sesame broccoli. Place broccoli florets on a separate baking sheet. Drizzle with olive oil and season with salt and pepper to taste. Toss to coat evenly.
7. Roast the broccoli in the oven for 10-12 minutes, or until tender-crisp and lightly browned.
8. Serve the ginger-soy glazed cod hot, with sesame broccoli and cooked rice or quinoa on the side.

Nutritional Information: (per serving, cod only)
- Calories: 200 kcal
- Carbohydrates: 10g
- Protein: 25g
- Fat: 7g
- Fiber: 2g

6. Magnesium-Packed Quinoa and Black Bean Stuffed Bell Peppers

Introduction: These magnesium-packed quinoa and black bean stuffed bell peppers are a nutritious and satisfying meal that's perfect for a meatless dinner option. Colorful bell peppers are filled with a flavorful mixture of quinoa, black beans, corn, and spices, then baked until tender for a delicious and protein-rich dish.

Total Prep Time: 45 minutes

Ingredients:
- 4 bell peppers (any color), halved and seeds removed
- 1 cup quinoa, rinsed
- 2 cups low-sodium vegetable broth
- 1 can (15 oz) black beans, drained and rinsed
- 1 cup corn kernels (fresh or frozen)
- 1 cup diced tomatoes (fresh or canned)
- 1 teaspoon ground cumin
- 1 teaspoon chili powder
- 1/2 teaspoon garlic powder
- Salt and pepper to taste
- Optional garnishes: chopped fresh cilantro, avocado slices, sour cream

Instructions:
1. Preheat the oven to 375°F (190°C). Grease a baking dish with cooking spray.
2. Place halved bell peppers in the prepared baking dish, cut side up.
3. In a saucepan, bring vegetable broth to a boil. Add rinsed quinoa and reduce heat to low. Cover and simmer for 15-20 minutes, or until quinoa is cooked and liquid is absorbed.
4. In a large mixing bowl, combine cooked quinoa, black beans, corn kernels, diced tomatoes, ground cumin, chili powder, garlic powder, salt, and pepper. Stir to combine.
5. Spoon the quinoa and black bean mixture evenly into the halved bell peppers, pressing down gently to pack the filling.
6. Cover the baking dish with aluminum foil and bake in the preheated oven for 25-30 minutes, or until the bell peppers are tender.
7. Remove the foil and bake for an additional 5 minutes, or until the tops are lightly browned.
8. Serve the magnesium-packed quinoa and black bean stuffed bell peppers hot, garnished with chopped fresh cilantro, avocado slices, and sour cream, if desired.

Dr. Lukas Loewe

Nutritional Information: (per serving, based on 1 stuffed bell pepper half)
- Calories: 200 kcal
- Carbohydrates: 35g
- Protein: 10g
- Fat: 3g
- Fiber: 7g

7. Ginger and Turmeric Roasted Chicken with Root Vegetables

Introduction: This ginger and turmeric roasted chicken with root vegetables is a wholesome and comforting meal that's perfect for a cozy dinner. Tender chicken thighs are marinated in a flavorful blend of ginger, turmeric, garlic, and herbs, then roasted to perfection alongside hearty root vegetables for a satisfying and nutritious dish.

Total Prep Time: 1 hour and 30 minutes

Ingredients:
- 4 chicken thighs, bone-in and skin-on
- 2 tablespoons olive oil
- 1 tablespoon freshly grated ginger
- 1 teaspoon ground turmeric
- 2 cloves garlic, minced
- 1 teaspoon dried thyme
- 1 teaspoon dried rosemary
- Salt and pepper to taste
- 2 large carrots, peeled and cut into chunks
- 2 parsnips, peeled and cut into chunks
- 1 sweet potato, peeled and cut into chunks
- 1 red onion, peeled and cut into wedges
- Fresh parsley for garnish

Instructions:
1. Preheat the oven to 400°F (200°C). Line a baking sheet with parchment paper.
2. In a small bowl, whisk together olive oil, freshly grated ginger, ground turmeric, minced garlic, dried thyme, dried rosemary, salt, and pepper to make the marinade.
3. Place chicken thighs in a large mixing bowl and pour the marinade over them. Toss to coat the chicken evenly with the marinade.

4. Arrange the marinated chicken thighs on one side of the prepared baking sheet.
5. In the same mixing bowl, toss chopped carrots, parsnips, sweet potato, and red onion with any remaining marinade.
6. Spread the seasoned root vegetables out on the other side of the baking sheet, making sure they are in a single layer.
7. Roast the chicken and vegetables in the preheated oven for 40-45 minutes, or until the chicken is cooked through and the vegetables are tender, stirring the vegetables halfway through cooking.
8. Once cooked, remove the baking sheet from the oven and let the chicken rest for a few minutes before serving.
9. Garnish the ginger and turmeric roasted chicken with root vegetables with fresh parsley before serving.

Nutritional Information: (per serving, based on 1 chicken thigh with vegetables)
- Calories: 350 kcal
- Carbohydrates: 20g
- Protein: 25g
- Fat: 18g
- Fiber: 5g

8. Magnesium-Rich Lentil and Kale Soup with Sausage

Introduction: This magnesium-rich lentil and kale soup with sausage is a hearty and nourishing dish that's perfect for a comforting meal. Packed with protein-rich lentils, nutritious kale, and flavorful sausage, this soup is seasoned with aromatic herbs and spices for a satisfying and flavorful bowl that will warm you from the inside out.

Total Prep Time: 1 hour

Ingredients:
- 1 cup dried green lentils, rinsed and drained
- 1 tablespoon olive oil
- 1 onion, diced
- 2 cloves garlic, minced
- 2 carrots, diced
- 2 celery stalks, diced
- 6 cups low-sodium chicken or vegetable broth
- 1 can (14 oz) diced tomatoes
- 2 cups chopped kale
- 8 oz cooked sausage, sliced

- 1 teaspoon dried thyme
- 1 teaspoon dried oregano
- Salt and pepper to taste
- Fresh parsley for garnish

Instructions:
1. In a large pot, heat olive oil over medium heat. Add diced onion and minced garlic, and sauté until softened and fragrant.
2. Add diced carrots and celery to the pot, and cook for an additional 5 minutes, until slightly softened.
3. Pour in low-sodium chicken or vegetable broth and bring the mixture to a boil.
4. Stir in rinsed and drained lentils, diced tomatoes (with their juices), dried thyme, dried oregano, salt, and pepper.
5. Reduce the heat to low, cover, and simmer for 30-40 minutes, or until the lentils are tender.
6. Add chopped kale and sliced cooked sausage to the pot, and simmer for an additional 10 minutes, until the kale is wilted and the sausage is heated through.
7. Adjust seasoning with salt and pepper to taste.
8. Serve the magnesium-rich lentil and kale soup hot, garnished with fresh parsley.

Nutritional Information: (per serving, based on 1 1/2 cups)
- Calories: 300 kcal
- Carbohydrates: 30g
- Protein: 15g
- Fat: 14g
- Fiber: 8g

9. Gingered Beef and Broccoli Stir-Fry with Brown Rice

Introduction: This gingered beef and broccoli stir-fry with brown rice is a wholesome and flavorful meal that's quick and easy to make. Tender strips of beef are stir-fried with crisp broccoli florets and aromatic ginger, then tossed in a savory sauce and served over nutritious brown rice for a satisfying dish that the whole family will love.

Total Prep Time: 30 minutes

Ingredients:
- 1 lb flank steak, thinly sliced against the grain
- 2 tablespoons soy sauce

- 1 tablespoon cornstarch
- 2 tablespoons vegetable oil
- 3 cloves garlic, minced
- 1 tablespoon freshly grated ginger
- 4 cups broccoli florets
- 1/4 cup low-sodium beef broth
- 2 tablespoons oyster sauce
- 1 tablespoon hoisin sauce
- Cooked brown rice for serving

Instructions:

1. In a bowl, combine thinly sliced flank steak with soy sauce and cornstarch. Toss to coat evenly and let marinate for 15-20 minutes.
2. Heat vegetable oil in a large skillet or wok over high heat.
3. Add minced garlic and freshly grated ginger to the skillet and cook for 1 minute, until fragrant.
4. Add marinated flank steak to the skillet in a single layer and cook for 2-3 minutes, until browned on all sides. Remove the beef from the skillet and set aside.
5. In the same skillet, add broccoli florets and stir-fry for 2-3 minutes, until crisp-tender.
6. Return the cooked beef to the skillet with the broccoli.
7. In a small bowl, whisk together low-sodium beef broth, oyster sauce, and hoisin sauce. Pour the sauce over the beef and broccoli in the skillet.
8. Stir-fry everything together for another minute, until heated through and evenly coated with the sauce.
9. Serve the gingered beef and broccoli stir-fry hot, over cooked brown rice.

Nutritional Information: (per serving, based on 4 servings)

- Calories: 350 kcal
- Carbohydrates: 20g
- Protein: 25g
- Fat: 18g
- Fiber: 4g

10. Magnesium-Boosting Chickpea and Spinach Masala with Naan Bread

Introduction: This magnesium-boosting chickpea and spinach masala with naan bread is a flavorful and nutritious dish that's perfect for a vegetarian dinner option. Creamy chickpeas are simmered in a fragrant tomato-based sauce with spinach and warm spices, then served alongside soft and fluffy naan bread for a satisfying meal that's full of flavor and goodness.

Total Prep Time: 40 minutes

Ingredients:
- 2 tablespoons vegetable oil
- 1 onion, finely chopped
- 3 cloves garlic, minced
- 1 tablespoon freshly grated ginger
- 1 teaspoon ground cumin
- 1 teaspoon ground coriander
- 1/2 teaspoon ground turmeric
- 1/2 teaspoon paprika
- 1/4 teaspoon cayenne pepper (optional, for heat)
- 1 can (15 oz) chickpeas, drained and rinsed
- 1 can (14 oz) diced tomatoes
- 2 cups baby spinach leaves
- 1/4 cup chopped fresh cilantro
- Salt and pepper to taste
- Store-bought or homemade naan bread for serving

Instructions:
1. Heat vegetable oil in a large skillet or pot over medium heat.
2. Add finely chopped onion to the skillet and cook for 5-6 minutes, until softened and translucent.
3. Stir in minced garlic and freshly grated ginger, and cook for another minute, until fragrant.
4. Add ground cumin, ground coriander, ground turmeric, paprika, and cayenne pepper (if using) to the skillet. Stir to combine with the onion mixture and cook for 1-2 minutes, until spices are toasted.
5. Add drained and rinsed chickpeas and diced tomatoes (with their juices) to the skillet. Stir to combine.
6. Reduce the heat to low and let the mixture simmer, uncovered, for 15-20 minutes, stirring occasionally, until the sauce has thickened slightly.
7. Stir in baby spinach leaves and chopped fresh cilantro, and cook for another 2-3 minutes, until the spinach wilts.
8. Season the chickpea and spinach masala with salt and pepper to taste.

9. Serve the magnesium-boosting chickpea and spinach masala hot, with warm naan bread for dipping and scooping.

Nutritional Information: (per serving, based on 4 servings, excluding naan bread)

- Calories: 250 kcal
- Carbohydrates: 30g
- Protein: 10g
- Fat: 10g
- Fiber: 8g

11. Ginger and Garlic Glazed Pork Tenderloin with Roasted Sweet Potatoes

Introduction: This ginger and garlic glazed pork tenderloin with roasted sweet potatoes is a delicious and satisfying meal that's perfect for a special dinner. Tender pork tenderloin is marinated in a flavorful ginger and garlic glaze, then roasted to perfection alongside sweet potatoes for a dish that's bursting with flavor and nutrients.

Total Prep Time: 1 hour and 15 minutes

Ingredients:

- 1 pork tenderloin (about 1 lb)
- 2 tablespoons olive oil
- 2 tablespoons soy sauce
- 2 tablespoons honey or maple syrup
- 1 tablespoon freshly grated ginger
- 2 cloves garlic, minced
- 1 teaspoon Dijon mustard
- Salt and pepper to taste
- 2 large sweet potatoes, peeled and cut into cubes
- Fresh parsley for garnish

Instructions:

1. Preheat the oven to 400°F (200°C). Line a baking sheet with parchment paper.
2. In a small bowl, whisk together olive oil, soy sauce, honey or maple syrup, freshly grated ginger, minced garlic, Dijon mustard, salt, and pepper to make the glaze.
3. Place the pork tenderloin on the prepared baking sheet. Brush the glaze over the pork, coating it evenly.

Dr. Lukas Loewe

4. In a separate bowl, toss cubed sweet potatoes with a drizzle of olive oil and a pinch of salt and pepper.
5. Arrange the sweet potatoes around the pork tenderloin on the baking sheet.
6. Roast in the preheated oven for 25-30 minutes, or until the pork is cooked through and the sweet potatoes are tender, flipping the sweet potatoes halfway through cooking.
7. Once cooked, remove the baking sheet from the oven and let the pork rest for a few minutes before slicing.
8. Slice the ginger and garlic glazed pork tenderloin and serve hot, with roasted sweet potatoes on the side.
9. Garnish with fresh parsley before serving.

Nutritional Information: (per serving, based on 4 servings)
- Calories: 300 kcal
- Carbohydrates: 25g
- Protein: 25g
- Fat: 10g
- Fiber: 3g

12. Magnesium-Rich Mediterranean Stuffed Zucchini with Quinoa and Feta

Introduction: These magnesium-rich Mediterranean stuffed zucchini boats are a delicious and nutritious way to enjoy seasonal produce. Tender zucchini halves are filled with a savory mixture of cooked quinoa, sun-dried tomatoes, olives, and feta cheese, then baked until golden and bubbly for a satisfying vegetarian meal.

Total Prep Time: 1 hour

Ingredients:
- 4 large zucchini
- 1 cup cooked quinoa
- 1/4 cup chopped sun-dried tomatoes
- 1/4 cup chopped Kalamata olives
- 1/4 cup crumbled feta cheese
- 2 tablespoons chopped fresh parsley
- 2 tablespoons olive oil
- 2 cloves garlic, minced
- Salt and pepper to taste
- Optional: grated Parmesan cheese for topping

Instructions:

1. Preheat the oven to 375°F (190°C). Line a baking dish with parchment paper.
2. Cut the zucchini in half lengthwise and use a spoon to scoop out the flesh, leaving about 1/4 inch border around the edges. Reserve the flesh for later use.
3. In a large mixing bowl, combine cooked quinoa, chopped sun-dried tomatoes, chopped Kalamata olives, crumbled feta cheese, chopped fresh parsley, olive oil, minced garlic, salt, and pepper. Mix well to combine.
4. Spoon the quinoa mixture into the hollowed-out zucchini halves, pressing down gently to pack the filling.
5. Place the stuffed zucchini boats in the prepared baking dish.
6. If desired, sprinkle grated Parmesan cheese over the top of each stuffed zucchini boat.
7. Bake in the preheated oven for 25-30 minutes, or until the zucchini is tender and the filling is heated through and lightly browned on top.
8. Remove from the oven and let cool for a few minutes before serving.
9. Serve the magnesium-rich Mediterranean stuffed zucchini hot, garnished with additional chopped parsley, if desired.

Nutritional Information: (per serving, based on 1 stuffed zucchini half)

- Calories: 180 kcal
- Carbohydrates: 15g
- Protein: 5g
- Fat: 10g
- Fiber: 3g

13. Ginger-Teriyaki Tofu Stir-Fry with Vegetables and Rice Noodles

Introduction: This ginger-teriyaki tofu stir-fry with vegetables and rice noodles is a flavorful and satisfying dish that's perfect for a quick and easy weeknight dinner. Crispy tofu cubes are tossed in a tangy ginger-teriyaki sauce, then stir-fried with colorful vegetables and tender rice noodles for a delicious and wholesome meal that's sure to please everyone at the table.

Total Prep Time: 30 minutes

Ingredients:
- 8 oz rice noodles
- 1 block (14 oz) firm tofu, drained and pressed
- 2 tablespoons soy sauce
- 2 tablespoons rice vinegar
- 1 tablespoon honey or maple syrup
- 1 tablespoon freshly grated ginger
- 2 cloves garlic, minced
- 2 tablespoons sesame oil, divided
- 1 red bell pepper, thinly sliced
- 1 yellow bell pepper, thinly sliced
- 1 cup snow peas, trimmed
- 1 carrot, julienned
- 2 green onions, sliced
- Sesame seeds for garnish
- Optional: chopped cilantro for garnish

Instructions:
1. Cook rice noodles according to package instructions until al dente. Drain and set aside.
2. While the noodles are cooking, prepare the tofu. Cut the pressed tofu into cubes and place them in a bowl.
3. In a small bowl, whisk together soy sauce, rice vinegar, honey or maple syrup, freshly grated ginger, minced garlic, and 1 tablespoon of sesame oil to make the sauce.
4. Pour half of the sauce over the tofu cubes and toss to coat evenly.
5. Heat the remaining tablespoon of sesame oil in a large skillet or wok over medium-high heat.
6. Add the marinated tofu cubes to the skillet in a single layer and cook for 3-4 minutes on each side, or until crispy and golden brown. Remove from the skillet and set aside.
7. In the same skillet, add sliced red bell pepper, sliced yellow bell pepper, snow peas, and julienned carrot. Stir-fry for 2-3 minutes, or until vegetables are tender-crisp.
8. Add cooked rice noodles, cooked tofu cubes, and remaining sauce to the skillet. Toss everything together until well combined and heated through.
9. Remove from heat and garnish with sliced green onions, sesame seeds, and chopped cilantro, if desired.

10. Serve the ginger-teriyaki tofu stir-fry hot, with additional soy sauce or chili sauce on the side, if desired.

Nutritional Information: (per serving)
- Calories: 350 kcal
- Carbohydrates: 50g
- Protein: 12g
- Fat: 12g
- Fiber: 6g

13. Ginger-Teriyaki Tofu Stir-Fry with Vegetables and Rice Noodles

Introduction: This ginger-teriyaki tofu stir-fry with vegetables and rice noodles is a flavorful and satisfying vegetarian dish that's quick and easy to make. Crispy tofu cubes are stir-fried with colorful vegetables and tender rice noodles, then tossed in a homemade ginger-teriyaki sauce for a delicious meal that's packed with flavor and nutrients.

Total Prep Time: 30 minutes

Ingredients:
- 8 oz rice noodles
- 1 block (14 oz) extra-firm tofu, drained and pressed
- 2 tablespoons soy sauce
- 1 tablespoon cornstarch
- 2 tablespoons vegetable oil, divided
- 2 cloves garlic, minced
- 1 tablespoon freshly grated ginger
- 2 cups mixed vegetables (such as bell peppers, snap peas, carrots, and broccoli)
- 1/4 cup low-sodium soy sauce
- 2 tablespoons hoisin sauce
- 1 tablespoon rice vinegar
- 1 tablespoon honey or maple syrup
- 1 teaspoon sesame oil
- Sesame seeds and sliced green onions for garnish

Instructions:
1. Cook rice noodles according to package instructions until al dente. Drain and set aside.
2. While the noodles are cooking, prepare the tofu. Cut the pressed tofu into cubes and pat dry with paper towels.

3. In a bowl, toss tofu cubes with soy sauce and cornstarch until evenly coated.
4. Heat 1 tablespoon of vegetable oil in a large skillet or wok over medium-high heat.
5. Add tofu cubes to the skillet in a single layer and cook for 4-5 minutes on each side, until golden and crispy. Remove tofu from the skillet and set aside.
6. In the same skillet, heat the remaining tablespoon of vegetable oil over medium heat.
7. Add minced garlic and freshly grated ginger to the skillet and cook for 1 minute, until fragrant.
8. Add mixed vegetables to the skillet and stir-fry for 3-4 minutes, until crisp-tender.
9. In a small bowl, whisk together low-sodium soy sauce, hoisin sauce, rice vinegar, honey or maple syrup, and sesame oil to make the ginger-teriyaki sauce.
10. Return the cooked tofu cubes to the skillet with the vegetables. Pour the ginger-teriyaki sauce over the tofu and vegetables, and toss to coat evenly.
11. Add the cooked rice noodles to the skillet and gently toss everything together until heated through.
12. Serve the ginger-teriyaki tofu stir-fry hot, garnished with sesame seeds and sliced green onions.

Nutritional Information: (per serving, based on 4 servings)
- Calories: 350 kcal
- Carbohydrates: 45g
- Protein: 12g
- Fat: 14g
- Fiber: 5g

14. Magnesium-Infused Spaghetti Squash Pad Thai with Shrimp

Introduction: This magnesium-infused spaghetti squash pad thai with shrimp is a healthy and flavorful twist on the classic Thai dish. Tender strands of spaghetti squash are tossed in a tangy and savory sauce, then topped with plump shrimp, crunchy peanuts, and fresh herbs for a delicious and nutritious meal that's sure to satisfy.

Total Prep Time: 1 hour

Ingredients:

- 1 medium spaghetti squash
- 1 tablespoon vegetable oil
- 1 lb shrimp, peeled and deveined
- 2 cloves garlic, minced
- 1 tablespoon freshly grated ginger
- 2 eggs, beaten
- 1 cup bean sprouts
- 1/4 cup chopped green onions
- 1/4 cup chopped cilantro
- 1/4 cup chopped roasted peanuts
- Lime wedges for serving

For the Pad Thai Sauce:

- 1/4 cup low-sodium soy sauce
- 2 tablespoons fish sauce
- 2 tablespoons rice vinegar
- 2 tablespoons lime juice
- 2 tablespoons honey or maple syrup
- 1 tablespoon sriracha (adjust to taste)
- 1 teaspoon sesame oil

Instructions:

1. Preheat the oven to 400°F (200°C). Cut the spaghetti squash in half lengthwise and scoop out the seeds. Place the squash halves, cut side down, on a baking sheet lined with parchment paper. Roast in the preheated oven for 40-50 minutes, or until the squash is tender and easily pierced with a fork. Once cooked, use a fork to scrape the flesh into spaghetti-like strands and set aside.
2. In a small bowl, whisk together all the ingredients for the pad thai sauce until well combined. Set aside.
3. In a large skillet or wok, heat vegetable oil over medium-high heat. Add minced garlic and grated ginger, and cook for 1 minute until fragrant.
4. Add the peeled and deveined shrimp to the skillet and cook for 2-3 minutes per side, until pink and cooked through. Remove the shrimp from the skillet and set aside.
5. Push the cooked shrimp to one side of the skillet and pour the beaten eggs into the other side. Scramble the eggs until cooked through, then mix them together with the shrimp.

6. Add the cooked spaghetti squash strands to the skillet along with the prepared pad thai sauce. Toss everything together until well combined and heated through.
7. Add bean sprouts and chopped green onions to the skillet and toss to combine.
8. Remove the skillet from heat and sprinkle chopped cilantro and roasted peanuts over the top.
9. Serve the magnesium-infused spaghetti squash pad thai with shrimp hot, garnished with lime wedges for squeezing over the top.

Nutritional Information: (per serving, based on 4 servings)
- Calories: 300 kcal
- Carbohydrates: 30g
- Protein: 25g
- Fat: 10g
- Fiber: 5g

15. Ginger-Lime Grilled Swordfish with Mango Salsa

Introduction: This ginger-lime grilled swordfish with mango salsa is a vibrant and flavorful dish that's perfect for summer grilling. Succulent swordfish steaks are marinated in a zesty ginger and lime marinade, then grilled to perfection and served with a refreshing mango salsa for a delicious and nutritious meal that's bursting with tropical flavors.

Total Prep Time: 30 minutes

Ingredients:
- 4 swordfish steaks (6 oz each)
- 2 tablespoons olive oil
- 2 tablespoons freshly squeezed lime juice
- 1 tablespoon freshly grated ginger
- 2 cloves garlic, minced
- 1 teaspoon honey or maple syrup
- Salt and pepper to taste

For the Mango Salsa:
- 1 ripe mango, peeled and diced
- 1/2 red bell pepper, diced
- 1/4 cup diced red onion
- 2 tablespoons chopped fresh cilantro
- 1 tablespoon freshly squeezed lime juice
- Salt and pepper to taste

Instructions:

1. In a small bowl, whisk together olive oil, lime juice, freshly grated ginger, minced garlic, honey or maple syrup, salt, and pepper to make the marinade.
2. Place swordfish steaks in a shallow dish and pour the marinade over them, turning to coat evenly. Cover and refrigerate for at least 15-20 minutes to marinate.
3. While the swordfish is marinating, prepare the mango salsa. In a medium bowl, combine diced mango, diced red bell pepper, diced red onion, chopped fresh cilantro, lime juice, salt, and pepper. Toss to combine and set aside.
4. Preheat the grill to medium-high heat. Lightly oil the grill grates to prevent sticking.
5. Remove swordfish steaks from the marinade and discard any excess marinade. Place the swordfish steaks on the preheated grill and cook for 4-5 minutes per side, or until the fish is cooked through and easily flakes with a fork.
6. Once cooked, remove the swordfish steaks from the grill and transfer to serving plates.
7. Serve the grilled swordfish hot, topped with a generous spoonful of mango salsa.

Nutritional Information: (per serving, based on 1 swordfish steak with mango salsa)

- Calories: 300 kcal
- Carbohydrates: 20g
- Protein: 25g
- Fat: 12g
- Fiber: 3g

16. Magnesium-Packed Moroccan Chickpea Stew with Couscous

Introduction: This magnesium-packed Moroccan chickpea stew with couscous is a flavorful and hearty dish inspired by the vibrant flavors of North African cuisine. Tender chickpeas are simmered in a fragrant tomato-based broth with warming spices, then served over fluffy couscous for a comforting and nutritious meal that's perfect for any occasion.

Total Prep Time: 1 hour and 15 minutes

Ingredients:

- 1 tablespoon olive oil

- 1 onion, diced
- 2 cloves garlic, minced
- 1 tablespoon freshly grated ginger
- 1 teaspoon ground cumin
- 1 teaspoon ground coriander
- 1/2 teaspoon ground cinnamon
- 1/4 teaspoon ground turmeric
- 1/4 teaspoon cayenne pepper (optional, for heat)
- 1 can (15 oz) chickpeas, drained and rinsed
- 1 can (14 oz) diced tomatoes
- 3 cups vegetable broth
- 1 cup diced carrots
- 1 cup diced sweet potatoes
- 1/4 cup chopped dried apricots
- Salt and pepper to taste
- Cooked couscous for serving
- Fresh cilantro for garnish

Instructions:

1. In a large pot, heat olive oil over medium heat. Add diced onion and cook for 5-6 minutes, until softened and translucent.
2. Add minced garlic and freshly grated ginger to the pot, and cook for another minute, until fragrant.
3. Stir in ground cumin, ground coriander, ground cinnamon, ground turmeric, and cayenne pepper (if using). Cook for 1-2 minutes, until spices are toasted.
4. Add drained and rinsed chickpeas, diced tomatoes (with their juices), vegetable broth, diced carrots, diced sweet potatoes, and chopped dried apricots to the pot. Stir to combine.
5. Bring the stew to a boil, then reduce the heat to low and let it simmer, covered, for 45-50 minutes, stirring occasionally, until the vegetables are tender and the flavors have melded together.
6. Season the stew with salt and pepper to taste.
7. Serve the magnesium-packed Moroccan chickpea stew hot, over cooked couscous.
8. Garnish with fresh cilantro before serving.

Nutritional Information: (per serving, based on 4 servings, excluding couscous)

- Calories: 250 kcal
- Carbohydrates: 40g
- Protein: 8g
- Fat: 6g
- Fiber: 8g

17. Ginger-Coconut Curry Tofu with Cauliflower Rice

Introduction: This ginger-coconut curry tofu with cauliflower rice is a flavorful and satisfying vegan dish that's perfect for a cozy dinner. Cubes of tofu are simmered in a creamy coconut curry sauce infused with aromatic ginger and warm spices, then served over nutritious cauliflower rice for a wholesome meal that's bursting with flavor and goodness.

Total Prep Time: 45 minutes

Ingredients:

- 1 block (14 oz) firm tofu, drained and pressed
- 2 tablespoons vegetable oil
- 1 onion, diced
- 2 cloves garlic, minced
- 1 tablespoon freshly grated ginger
- 2 tablespoons red curry paste
- 1 can (14 oz) coconut milk
- 1 tablespoon soy sauce
- 1 tablespoon maple syrup or brown sugar
- 1 teaspoon ground turmeric
- 1/2 teaspoon ground coriander
- 1/4 teaspoon cayenne pepper (optional, for heat)
- Salt and pepper to taste
- 1 small head cauliflower, grated into rice-like texture
- Chopped fresh cilantro for garnish
- Lime wedges for serving

Instructions:

1. Cut the pressed tofu into cubes and set aside.
2. In a large skillet or pot, heat vegetable oil over medium heat. Add diced onion and cook for 5-6 minutes, until softened and translucent.
3. Add minced garlic and freshly grated ginger to the skillet, and cook for another minute, until fragrant.
4. Stir in red curry paste and cook for 1-2 minutes, until fragrant.

5. Pour in coconut milk, soy sauce, maple syrup or brown sugar, ground turmeric, ground coriander, and cayenne pepper (if using). Stir to combine.
6. Add tofu cubes to the skillet and gently stir to coat with the curry sauce. Let the mixture simmer for 10-12 minutes, stirring occasionally, until the tofu is heated through and the sauce has thickened slightly.
7. While the tofu is simmering, prepare the cauliflower rice. Grate the cauliflower into a rice-like texture using a box grater or food processor.
8. Heat a separate skillet over medium heat and add the grated cauliflower. Cook for 5-6 minutes, stirring occasionally, until the cauliflower is tender and heated through. Season with salt and pepper to taste.
9. Serve the ginger-coconut curry tofu hot, over cauliflower rice.
10. Garnish with chopped fresh cilantro and serve with lime wedges on the side.

Nutritional Information: (per serving, based on 4 servings)
- Calories: 300 kcal
- Carbohydrates: 15g
- Protein: 10g
- Fat: 25g
- Fiber: 5g

17. Ginger-Coconut Curry Tofu with Cauliflower Rice

Introduction: This ginger-coconut curry tofu with cauliflower rice is a delicious and satisfying vegan dish that's packed with flavor and nutrients. Crispy tofu cubes are simmered in a creamy coconut curry sauce infused with ginger and spices, then served over fluffy cauliflower rice for a low-carb alternative to traditional rice. It's a wholesome and comforting meal that's perfect for any day of the week.

Total Prep Time: 40 minutes

Ingredients:
- 1 block (14 oz) extra-firm tofu, drained and pressed
- 2 tablespoons vegetable oil, divided
- 1 onion, diced
- 3 cloves garlic, minced
- 1 tablespoon freshly grated ginger

- 1 tablespoon curry powder
- 1 teaspoon ground turmeric
- 1/2 teaspoon ground cumin
- 1 can (14 oz) coconut milk
- 1 tablespoon soy sauce or tamari
- 1 tablespoon maple syrup or coconut sugar
- Salt and pepper to taste
- 1 head cauliflower, riced (or store-bought cauliflower rice)
- Fresh cilantro for garnish

Instructions:

1. Cut the pressed tofu into cubes and pat dry with paper towels.
2. Heat 1 tablespoon of vegetable oil in a large skillet or wok over medium-high heat. Add the tofu cubes to the skillet in a single layer and cook for 4-5 minutes on each side, until golden and crispy. Remove tofu from the skillet and set aside.
3. In the same skillet, heat the remaining tablespoon of vegetable oil over medium heat. Add diced onion and cook for 5-6 minutes, until softened and translucent.
4. Add minced garlic and freshly grated ginger to the skillet and cook for another minute, until fragrant.
5. Stir in curry powder, ground turmeric, and ground cumin, and cook for 1-2 minutes, until spices are toasted.
6. Pour coconut milk into the skillet and stir to combine with the onion and spice mixture.
7. Add soy sauce or tamari, maple syrup or coconut sugar, salt, and pepper to taste. Stir to combine.
8. Return the cooked tofu cubes to the skillet and let the curry simmer for 10-15 minutes, until the sauce has thickened slightly.
9. While the curry is simmering, prepare the cauliflower rice. If using a head of cauliflower, chop it into florets and pulse in a food processor until it resembles rice-like grains.
10. Serve the ginger-coconut curry tofu hot, over cauliflower rice.
11. Garnish with fresh cilantro before serving.

Nutritional Information: (per serving, based on 4 servings, excluding cauliflower rice)

- Calories: 300 kcal

- Carbohydrates: 10g
- Protein: 10g
- Fat: 25g
- Fiber: 2g

18. Magnesium-Rich Turkey and Vegetable Chili with Beans

Introduction: This magnesium-rich turkey and vegetable chili with beans is a hearty and nutritious meal that's perfect for chilly days. Lean ground turkey is simmered with a variety of colorful vegetables, beans, and warming spices to create a flavorful and satisfying dish that the whole family will love. It's easy to make, packed with protein and fiber, and full of essential nutrients to keep you feeling energized and satisfied.

Total Prep Time: 1 hour and 15 minutes

Ingredients:

- 1 tablespoon olive oil
- 1 onion, diced
- 2 cloves garlic, minced
- 1 red bell pepper, diced
- 1 green bell pepper, diced
- 1 jalapeño pepper, seeded and diced
- 1 lb lean ground turkey
- 1 can (14 oz) diced tomatoes
- 1 can (15 oz) kidney beans, drained and rinsed
- 1 can (15 oz) black beans, drained and rinsed
- 2 cups vegetable broth
- 2 tablespoons tomato paste
- 2 teaspoons chili powder
- 1 teaspoon ground cumin
- 1 teaspoon smoked paprika
- Salt and pepper to taste
- Fresh cilantro for garnish
- Optional toppings: shredded cheese, sour cream, avocado slices, diced green onions

Instructions:

1. Heat olive oil in a large pot over medium heat. Add diced onion, minced garlic, diced red bell pepper, diced green bell pepper, and diced jalapeño pepper to the pot. Cook for

5-6 minutes, stirring occasionally, until vegetables are softened.

2. Add lean ground turkey to the pot and cook, breaking it apart with a spoon, until browned and cooked through.
3. Stir in diced tomatoes (with their juices), drained and rinsed kidney beans, drained and rinsed black beans, vegetable broth, tomato paste, chili powder, ground cumin, smoked paprika, salt, and pepper.
4. Bring the chili to a simmer, then reduce the heat to low and let it simmer, uncovered, for 45-50 minutes, stirring occasionally, to allow the flavors to meld together and the chili to thicken.
5. Taste and adjust seasoning with salt and pepper as needed.
6. Serve the magnesium-rich turkey and vegetable chili hot, garnished with fresh cilantro and your choice of optional toppings.

Nutritional Information: (per serving, based on 6 servings)
- Calories: 300 kcal
- Carbohydrates: 30g
- Protein: 25g
- Fat: 10g
- Fiber: 10g

19. Ginger and Garlic Glazed Beef Skewers with Grilled Vegetables

Introduction: These ginger and garlic glazed beef skewers with grilled vegetables are a delicious and flavorful dish that's perfect for summer grilling. Tender chunks of beef are marinated in a zesty ginger and garlic marinade, then threaded onto skewers with colorful vegetables and grilled to perfection. The result is a mouthwatering meal that's sure to impress your family and friends at your next barbecue.

Total Prep Time: 1 hour and 30 minutes (including marinating time)

Ingredients:
- 1 lb beef sirloin or flank steak, cut into 1-inch cubes
- 2 bell peppers (any color), cut into 1-inch pieces
- 1 red onion, cut into 1-inch pieces
- Cherry tomatoes

- Wooden or metal skewers
- Fresh cilantro for garnish

For the Ginger and Garlic Glaze:

- 3 tablespoons soy sauce
- 2 tablespoons honey or maple syrup
- 2 tablespoons rice vinegar
- 1 tablespoon freshly grated ginger
- 2 cloves garlic, minced
- 1 teaspoon sesame oil
- Salt and pepper to taste

Instructions:

1. If using wooden skewers, soak them in water for at least 30 minutes to prevent them from burning on the grill.
2. In a small bowl, whisk together soy sauce, honey or maple syrup, rice vinegar, freshly grated ginger, minced garlic, sesame oil, salt, and pepper to make the ginger and garlic glaze.
3. Place the cubed beef in a shallow dish or resealable plastic bag. Pour the ginger and garlic glaze over the beef, ensuring it is evenly coated. Cover or seal and refrigerate for at least 1 hour, or overnight, to marinate.
4. Preheat the grill to medium-high heat. Lightly oil the grill grates to prevent sticking.
5. Thread marinated beef cubes onto skewers, alternating with bell pepper pieces, red onion pieces, and cherry tomatoes.
6. Place the assembled skewers on the preheated grill and cook for 8-10 minutes, turning occasionally, until the beef is cooked to your desired level of doneness and the vegetables are tender and slightly charred.
7. Remove the skewers from the grill and transfer to a serving platter.
8. Garnish the ginger and garlic glazed beef skewers with fresh cilantro before serving.

Nutritional Information: (per serving, based on 4 servings)

- Calories: 250 kcal
- Carbohydrates: 15g
- Protein: 25g
- Fat: 10g
- Fiber: 3g

20. Magnesium-Boosting Lemon-Ginger Baked Cod with Asparagus

Introduction: This magnesium-boosting lemon-ginger baked cod with asparagus is a light and flavorful dish that's perfect for a healthy weeknight dinner. Tender cod fillets are marinated in a zesty lemon and ginger marinade, then baked to perfection alongside fresh asparagus spears for a nutritious and delicious meal that's quick and easy to prepare.

Total Prep Time: 30 minutes

Ingredients:
- 4 cod fillets (about 6 oz each)
- 1 lb asparagus, trimmed
- 2 tablespoons olive oil
- 2 tablespoons freshly squeezed lemon juice
- 1 tablespoon freshly grated ginger
- 2 cloves garlic, minced
- 1 teaspoon lemon zest
- Salt and pepper to taste
- Fresh parsley for garnish
- Lemon wedges for serving

Instructions:
1. Preheat the oven to 400°F (200°C). Line a baking sheet with parchment paper or foil.
2. In a small bowl, whisk together olive oil, lemon juice, freshly grated ginger, minced garlic, lemon zest, salt, and pepper to make the marinade.
3. Place cod fillets and trimmed asparagus spears on the prepared baking sheet.
4. Pour the marinade over the cod fillets and asparagus, ensuring they are evenly coated.
5. Let the cod and asparagus marinate for 15-20 minutes at room temperature.
6. Once marinated, transfer the baking sheet to the preheated oven and bake for 12-15 minutes, or until the cod is opaque and flakes easily with a fork, and the asparagus is tender.
7. Remove the baking sheet from the oven and transfer the baked cod and asparagus to serving plates.

8. Garnish with fresh parsley and serve with lemon wedges on the side.

Nutritional Information: (per serving, based on 4 servings)
- Calories: 200 kcal
- Carbohydrates: 6g
- Protein: 25g
- Fat: 8g
- Fiber: 3g

6.4 1-Week Meal Plan

Sunday:
Breakfast: Ginger-infused Oatmeal with Almonds and Honey
Lunch: Grilled Chicken and Ginger Stir-Fry with Broccoli and Bell Peppers
Dinner: Ginger and Garlic Shrimp Stir-Fry with Snow Peas and Bell Peppers

Monday:
Breakfast: Magnesium-Rich Spinach and Feta Omelette
Lunch: Magnesium-Rich Quinoa Salad with Chickpeas and Roasted Vegetables
Dinner: Magnesium-Rich Baked Salmon with Lemon and Dill

Tuesday:
Breakfast: Gingerbread Pancakes with Maple Syrup
Lunch: Ginger-Lime Shrimp Tacos with Mango Salsa
Dinner: Ginger-Coconut Chicken Curry with Jasmine Rice

Wednesday:
Breakfast: Mango-Ginger Smoothie with Chia Seeds
Lunch: Magnesium-Packed Lentil Soup with Spinach and Turmeric
Dinner: Magnesium-Infused Vegetable Stir-Fry with Tofu

Thursday:
Breakfast: Avocado Toast with Smoked Salmon and Pickled Ginger

Lunch: Ginger and Garlic Tofu Stir-Fry with Brown Rice
Dinner: Ginger-Soy Glazed Cod with Sesame Broccoli

Friday:
Breakfast: Turmeric-Ginger Overnight Oats with Berries
Lunch: Magnesium-Boosting Greek Salad with Feta and Kalamata Olives
Dinner: Magnesium-Packed Quinoa and Black Bean Stuffed Bell Peppers

Saturday:
Breakfast: Magnesium-Boosting Banana Walnut Muffins
Lunch: Ginger-Soy Glazed Salmon Salad with Avocado and Edamame
Dinner: Ginger and Turmeric Roasted Chicken with Root Vegetables

This meal plan offers a variety of delicious and nutritious meals throughout the week, incorporating the provided recipes for breakfast, lunch, and dinner. Each day features a balance of flavors and nutrients, ensuring a satisfying and well-rounded culinary experience. Enjoy your week of healthy eating!

CHAPTER 7:
CONCLUSION

In conclusion, "Ginger and Magnesium Book" A Culinary Journey to Holistic Wellness" offers readers a unique and transformative exploration of well-being that seamlessly integrates science, tradition, and the pleasure of delicious, nutritious meals. As we navigate the pages of this book, we discover not only the incredible health benefits of ginger and magnesium but also a culinary adventure that turns healthy eating into a flavorful and enjoyable experience.

The fusion of ginger and magnesium emerges as a dynamic duo, unlocking a world of possibilities for those seeking a holistic approach to their health. This book goes beyond mere information; it becomes a companion in the kitchen, guiding readers to harness the power of these elements through a curated selection of healthy, nutritious, and delectable recipes.

Ginger, with its aromatic warmth and versatile profile, takes center stage in a series of culinary creations that extend far beyond the conventional. From zesty ginger-infused salads to comforting soups and invigorating smoothies, each recipe is crafted to showcase the culinary prowess of this superfood. By incorporating ginger into our daily meals, we not only elevate the taste but also infuse our bodies with its anti-inflammatory and digestive benefits.

Complementing the vibrant flavors of ginger, the inclusion of magnesium-rich ingredients in the recipes underscores the commitment of this book to a well-rounded and balanced approach to nutrition. Magnesium, often overlooked in traditional culinary narratives, finds its place in these dishes, enhancing not only their taste but also contributing to the overall well-being of those who savor them.

One of the distinctive features of "Ginger and Magnesium Book" is the provision of a carefully crafted 1-week meal plan that seamlessly integrates these recipes into a practical and achievable routine. This meal plan is not a restrictive regimen but a flexible guide that accommodates various preferences and dietary needs. It is designed to simplify the often-daunting task of meal preparation, ensuring that readers can embark on their wellness journey with confidence and ease.

The beauty of the meal plan lies in its diversity and simplicity. Each day brings a delightful array of dishes, from hearty breakfasts to satisfying dinners, all designed to nourish the body and tantalize the taste buds. By incorporating the principles of balance and variety, the meal plan caters to the diverse palates and lifestyles of readers, making the pursuit of health an enjoyable and sustainable endeavor.

Furthermore, the inclusion of nutritional information alongside each recipe empowers readers to make informed choices about their dietary intake. Whether one is focused on weight management, energy enhancement, or specific health goals, this book provides the tools necessary to align culinary choices with individual wellness objectives.

Beyond the realm of recipes, "Ginger and Magnesium Book" fosters a deeper understanding of the intimate connection between food and well-being. The book delves into mindful eating practices, encouraging readers to savor each bite and appreciate the nourishment provided by the ingredients. This mindful approach extends beyond the kitchen, inviting readers to cultivate a holistic relationship with their food and, by extension, their overall health.

As we conclude our journey through the pages of "Ginger and Magnesium Book," we are left with a profound appreciation for the transformative potential that lies within our daily meals. This book transcends the conventional boundaries of a health guide; it becomes a culinary companion, a wellness coach, and a source of inspiration for those seeking a vibrant and fulfilling life.

In essence, "Ginger and Magnesium Book" is an invitation to not only read about but actively participate in the creation of a healthier, more balanced life. By embracing the synergy of ginger and magnesium in our kitchens, we embark on a delicious adventure that goes beyond nourishing the body; it nourishes the soul, transforming the act of eating into a celebration of well-being.